The LMNOPs of Surviving Cancer

Let Me Now Offer Praise!

Karla Heeter
Jan Heyerdahl

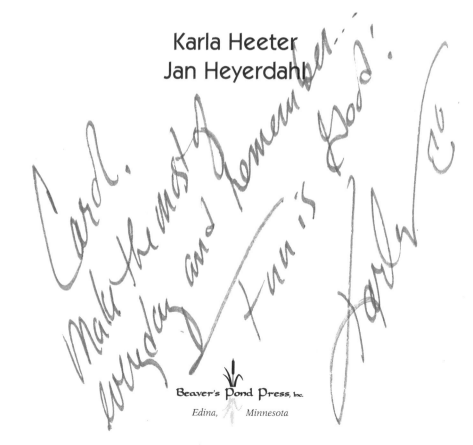

Beaver's Pond Press, Inc.
Edina, Minnesota

Special thanks to Holly Minke for editing our writings, and Ken Lunderby for his professional photography.

To help the people of Wright County, Minnesota "get a jump on cancer," part of the proceeds from the sale of each book will go to the Community Health Foundation of Wright County.

Production Supervisor: Milton Adams

ISBN 1-890676-00-00

Library of Congress Catalog Card Number: 00-107636

Printed in the United States of America

03 02 01 00 4 5 4 3 2 1

Dedications

Karla's Dedication:

To my husband and best friend, Ron, I will be forever grateful for your unconditional love, patience and support.

To my nieces and nephews, Mikey, Sarah, Mitchell, Julia, Olivia, Spencer and Tyler. May you love life and the Lord as much as I do!

And to my very special friend Jamie, who has taught me so many life lessons. One of the most important of those lessons is "If you have Jesus in your heart, then dying isn't a bad thing."

Jan's Dedication:

To my family whose love sustained me:

Steve, Paul, Chrissy and Mike, your strength became my strength.

Mom and Dad, you gave and continue to give me life, refreshing and renewing me with your love.

Tammy, your companionship has brought me light on my darkest days. Shine on, Sista!

To all of those who prayed for me, this book is for you!

Table of Contents

Authors' Note

Who are we to write about cancer? Who are we to tell others what to expect or what to do when they hear a diagnosis of cancer?

We've "been there, done that!" We are survivors!

Our **A**ttitudes, **B**eliefs and **C**hallenges, **R**eflections, **S**tories and **T**hanksgivings are simply stated, from **A** to **Z**, on the following pages. May our words bring you hope and inspiration.

Your investment in this book will help others, as part of the proceeds from the sale of each book will go to the Community Health Foundation of Wright County to help others "get a jump on cancer!"

Introduction

Karla's Story

In the Fall of 1996, at the age of 38, I began experiencing break-through bleeding between my periods. In addition, I was having a fair amount of lower abdominal, pelvic area discomfort. It could be compared to mild menstrual cramping or a nagging soreness. One might say I could "feel my female reproductive organs all the time."

As the holidays drew near, I was having an unusual vaginal discharge. It was not like that of an ovulation discharge, nor was it typical of a yeast infection. It was a wet, odorless discharge that left a dark film on the outer edges of the soiled area. I had to wear a sanitary pad around the clock to manage this inconvenient symptom.

Along with these symptoms that lead to my concern, I had, for a couple of years, a great deal of indigestion with some bloating and full feeling.

I called for a doctor's appointment in late January, and I was told that I could not get in to see my regular family physician for a couple of months. I then called him directly and asked what I might do in light of my situation and his full schedule. He referred me to the Women's Clinic on the lower level of his practice. They were booking several weeks out, so I set an appointment for early March.

When I arrived for this appointment, a very busy female Ob-Gyn doctor greeted me. She had an arm full of charts and not much time to hear about my symptoms and discomfort. She did a pelvic exam and Pap smear and sent me on my way, telling me "We'll just watch things for three months."

After a few weeks, I returned with no change in my situation. She then did a pelvic ultrasound, said my ovary was enlarged, but I shouldn't be too concerned. After all, she assured me, I was too young for cancer. She suggested I try some birth control pills for three months to see if this might "fix things."

After just a month on the pill, I called and asked to come in again as I was having a great deal of bleeding, discharge and discomfort. I knew this was not normal. Something was happening. My body was telling me to look further.

I arrived for this appointment and was greeted by an obviously fed up physician who proceeded to ask me a number of what I would call ridiculous questions. She asked, "Do you bleed when you jump up and down?" and "You don't suppose you're just leaking urine, do you?" It was apparent to me that she thought I was making too much of my symptoms, because again, I was "too young for cancer."

At this same visit, she scheduled me for an endometrial biopsy the next week. Scared to death of this simple procedure, I called my regular family physician and asked him for something to help me get back through the door for this upcoming appointment. I also asked that he look at my chart and give me feedback on my symptoms, the chain of events, etc. He did and assured me that this doctor was a great lady and that I should trust her judgment and findings.

My husband took off work early to accompany me to this endometrial biopsy appointment. I arrived, somewhat calm from the little yellow pill my family doc prescribed, ready to get this over with, behind me. I wanted some answers.

The nurse came in, took my blood pressure and was about to leave the room, when I asked her if I should undress. She said no, that the doctor wanted to talk to me first and she didn't think they were going to do the biopsy. I was puzzled, somewhat relieved; yet concerned that I'd still not have any answers.

The doctor came in 10-15 minutes later, her arm full of charts and one hand on the doorknob. She said that she'd reviewed my chart and thought that this biopsy was really not necessary. It was expensive, uncomfortable and she really didn't think we needed to do it at this time. She suggested I go home and call her in two to three months if I continued to have problems.

I left her office totally deflated, not knowing where I should turn. The next day, my hairdresser suggested that I see her Ob-Gyn, Dr. Linda Maag. This was my lucky day! I set an appointment with this new physician, and she would do an endometrial biopsy ON THE SPOT!

I received a phone call on June 9, 1997. My endometrial biopsy revealed uterine cancer. Surgery was scheduled for the next day. Ovarian cancer was found during the surgery. Chemotherapy followed. Three years later, I am a survivor!

A – Animals

For as long as I can remember, animals have played a big part in my life. The beauty of domesticated animals (cats and dogs) is that they love you unconditionally. When you're well, when you're sick, when you're happy and when you're sad, whether you have money or not, even if you have bad breath (especially when you have bad breath), animals love you. Animals give us reason to live, reason to get up and move; they depend on us for their care.

I never missed a day of choring my horses during chemotherapy. It was good therapy for me. Often I needed to sit on a bale of hay as the horses ate, and I regrouped and gained the strength I needed to nourish them. Caring for them on a daily basis was an important part of caring for me.

On the days when I was in bed, recuperating from chemotherapy, my two Whippets, Zipper and Kazoo, were right there by my side, hour after hour, keeping me warm and loved. Animals really do make our lives richer.

Affirmations

One day while surfin' the net for a meaningful quote to compliment a grant I was writing for the Community Health Foundation, I found this thought-provoking quote. I wanted to move the grant readers and thought an inspirational quote might be the answer. Although I did not use this quote for the grant, it moved me and has been etched in my memory ever since.

> **"Imagine you were given just a short time to live**
> **and you could make one phone call.**
> **Who would you call and what would you say...**
> **and what are you waiting for?"**

It's so simple, yet so profound...and it's so true. So often we wait until it's too late, never taking the opportunity to let people know how wonderful they are or that we love them. At work or home, with friends or with family, in all aspects of our lives, we need to seize the moment...let someone know you care!

After I read this quote, the first person that came to my mind was my dad, Bob. I know I've told him that I love him and that I think he's a wonderful man. He's not my biological father. Somebody else fathered me, but anyone could have done that. Bob is my dad. He was there for me. He raised me, fed me and clothed me. He cares!

I know he knows how grateful I am, but I'd like to say it again...Thanks, Dad! I Love You!

B – Bavarian Cancer

Just eight months after I had been diagnosed with Ovarian Cancer, my mother was seated at the center island in my kitchen complaining about pelvic area pain and discomfort when she was asked to post during her riding lessons. She complained of a bloated feeling and excess gas. I asked if she had any heartburn to which she replied, "for the last month or two, everything gives me heartburn." I told her that she was experiencing the classic symptoms of ovarian cancer.

She would see my Ob-Gyn, Dr. Maag, have a CA 125 test, a pelvic exam and a vaginal ultrasound. Her tumor was much larger than mine and initially appeared to be quite advanced.

After her surgery when the doctor told the family that she did indeed have ovarian cancer, my Dad pulled me aside and said, "What is Bavarian Cancer anyway?" I responded with a chuckle and asked him to repeat the question. I think he realized that he might be saying it wrong and came back saying, "Well Ballbarian cancer, what is that?"

To this day, we chuckle at Dad's lack of knowledge of the female reproductive system. In his day that was rarely ever the topic of conversation among couples. After all, he couldn't even go in the labor and delivery room when his daughter was born. My how the times have changed!

Mom survived. Her tumor was totally encapsulated, stage 1, with no metastases. She would not even require further treatment. What a miracle that we would both be diagnosed with the rarely heard of, *stage 1* ovarian cancer.

Bette

In surviving cancer, a good medical support team is imperative. A competent Ob-Gyn, surgeon and oncologist are important ingredients to survival. But who would ever guess that the person at the front desk, the one who greets you when you arrive at the clinic, takes your phone calls and makes your physician referrals, could have such an impact on your life.

My newfound friend, Bette, at the John A. Haugen and Associates Clinic gave me such strength and security. She made my doctor accessible to me, made all the medical processes easy and most importantly: she made me feel like I mattered. I was a priority, someone of value, not "just another patient." Bette knows how to take care of people. She knew and could sense when I needed hand holding.

Every clinic needs a Bette. All too often, in health care, we are greeted as and treated like a patient chart or a number. Medicine is about people not illness. It's unfortunate that the business of medicine gets in the way of the practice of caring about people.

I thank Bette for making it easy to come to the clinic and to call. She is key to my survival.

C – Chicken Divan

Chemo, for me, had a cumulative effect. After the first and second treatments I didn't get very sick, but I was pretty tired and in bed for the first couple of days. After chemo two, I actually vomited for the first time. But, after my third chemo whenever I would go to the hospital to stay for my 36-hour treatment, I would put a sign on my door saying, "No hospital food in this room." When they would pass food down the hall to other people, I could smell it. Even today if I go to visit someone in the hospital, the smell of hospital food sort of makes me feel a bit nauseated. This is, in no way, a judgment call on hospital food. The hospital food was quite good; I just couldn't stand the smell, so I asked that food not be brought into my room.

I don't know what the menu cycles are, but it seemed like every three weeks when I would come to the hospital, the Monday night choice was Chicken Divan. Now the first time or two I was there, I loved it. Chicken Divan is a wonderful chicken hot dish with white sauce and broccoli and it's usually really good.

After the second time I ate the Chicken Divan, I became nauseated so I didn't want anymore. But any time I would go to the hospital they would have Chicken Divan on the menu and that was the meal they would deliver to my room. It got so that I couldn't stand Chicken Divan. I mean the looks of it and the smell of it made me sick. And you know how broccoli smells when it's cooked, kind of nasty.

I went home after my fourth or fifth treatment and one of my dear friends and great supporters, Sandy Frank, stopped over at my house and brought me this wonderful warm dinner. I wasn't feeling very well so I set it on the counter, thanked her for everything and she left. I didn't even have to open the towel or lift the lid off this hot dish; I knew by the smell that it was Chicken Divan.

I put it in the fridge thinking that maybe tomorrow I'll be hungry. The next morning as I lay in bed, my husband was getting ready for work and opened the refrigerator to get milk for his cereal. I could smell the Chicken Divan from my bedroom more than 30 feet from the refrigerator. I called out to Ron, "The Chicken Divan has to go outside!" He said "What do you mean?" To which I replied, "The

Chicken Divan has to go outside. I can smell it way back here and you have to get it out of the house, I just can't have it in here!"

So, I had to throw it away. To this day, Sandy Frank, to this day doesn't know that I had to throw her Chicken Divan away. She will read about it in this book. Bless your heart Sandy for being so kind and thoughtful, your intentions were so good. I'M SORRY I THREW AWAY THE CHICKEN DIVAN. I know you worked hard and I am grateful to you for the kind gesture. No Chicken Divan at my house, not today or any other day.

Community Health Foundation of Wright County

The Community Health Foundation of Wright County was founded in 1983 for the purpose of giving back to the community to affect health-related needs and endeavors. In the Fall of 1996, the Foundation Board came together at a retreat to talk about how we might grow the organization and make a greater impact on the people of Wright County. As a result of this discussion, an Executive Director was hired to do a health-needs assessment and feasibility study. We wanted to find out who knows us, what they think of us and what the most emerging health need in the county might be.

We discovered two things. First, the Foundation was one of Wright County's best-kept secrets! People were unaware that in our first 15 years, the foundation had given away over $200,000! Unless people specifically knew someone on the board, they didn't know what the Foundation was all about.

We also learned that cancer is the number one health concern of people in Wright County. People are moved by cancer, concerned about cancer, and even fear cancer. Everyone knows someone whose life is touched by cancer...someone in the family, the community, in the workplace, in church…some who are beating cancer and some who are not. To that end, we created our project to help the people of Wright County: "The Wright Cancer Prescription!" Our purpose is to help people "get a jump on cancer" with education on cancer prevention and early detection.

Statistics tell us that 1 in 3 women and half of all men will experience cancer in their lifetime. We want to help people "get a jump on cancer" by hopping around the county with a pouch full of resources! Our kangaroo mascot is named Wrighty Roo. Kangaroos are healthy, active animals that eat a lot of greens and do not get cancer.

The morning of the very day that I was to have a 2:00 interview for the executive director position with Community Health Foundation, I received the phone call with my cancer diagnosis. How ironic that I should be diagnosed with cancer, have to withdraw as a candidate to lead the Foundation in order to fight cancer, and then become the Cancer Project Director. God had a plan! So often, we want to be in control and think that we know best, but the Father knows best! I thought I missed out on the best job opportunity of my career. The Lord knew there was other work for me to do…we must listen for the answer to our prayers!

D – Diagnosis Day

The date was June 9, 1997, a date that will be forever etched in my memory; probably long after I've forgotten my own wedding anniversary and birthday, I'll remember this day. I think, for other cancer survivors, this is probably one of the most significant days in their entire life.

On the day I received my diagnosis, I was scheduled to go to the Medical Arts Building in downtown Minneapolis at two o'clock in the afternoon for a vaginal ultrasound. I was spotting quite heavily that morning so at about 9:15 a.m., I called the clinic where I was supposed to go to let them know that I was indeed bleeding and asked if I should still come in for the procedure. They asked what time was my appointment, and I responded by saying I think 2:00 or 2:15. They looked in the book and asked my name and then said my appointment had been cancelled. They assumed that I had already cancelled it. I told them I had not and didn't understand who would have cancelled the appointment.

After more checking, they said my doctor had cancelled the appointment. I just assumed the results of my biopsy came back with no problems, so why do any further tests. I did not, for one moment, think about this being as serious as it was. I don't know what was going on in my head, but I wasn't even considering that I might have cancer.

I provide foster care for homeless and abandoned animals, and I was caring for a darling little collie puppy, named Callie, during this confusing call about the ultrasound. It wasn't even five minutes after my call to the Medical Arts building to see if I should come in, when my phone rang. It was Dr. Maag. She said that my biopsy results had come back and that she had indeed tried to reach me on Friday, could not get me and didn't want to leave this on my voice mail. As she was calling for me on that Friday, June 6th, I was at Buffalo High School all day long, chairing the All-Night Graduation Party. I arrived at the high school at 8:00 a.m. Friday and didn't return home until about 8:00 a.m. Saturday. Thank God, again! He always has a plan. He knows what's right. He knows about the timing and He just didn't allow me to know on that day. How could I have ever gotten through that night knowing I had cancer? That whole night would have ended up being, for my committee, about me. And that's not what it should have been.

The other thing that's really interesting about this is that after we had our Grad Party debriefing three weeks later, everyone said that I was on edge and that they knew something was going on. I don't remember feeling or being aware that it was weighing heavy on my mind.

When I got the call from Dr. Maag, she said she got the biopsy results back and tried to reach me on Friday but couldn't, and that she wanted to speak to me in person. She said, "I don't have very good news. The test results show that you have cancer." I just very sternly said, "OK, so what do we do now?" In a very matter of fact way she told me that I needed to have surgery. They got only a small amount of tissue in the endometrial biopsy, and there were a lot of cancer cells. She suggested that we do surgery the next day. Which, of course, scared me, but you must also know that she was due to have a baby in two weeks. She wanted to do the surgery with her partner, so she wanted us to move quickly. She had already checked and could get space in the operating room the next day. I said I was willing to do surgery then, and she wanted to know if I could be at her office before noon, for my pre-op exam.

I remember hanging the phone up and just covering my face with my hands and literally falling to the floor in tears. I thought, who do I call? What do I do? Here I had this interview with the Community Health Foundation later that day. So I hung up and I called my husband at work. I was just a mess. I look back, and I think I was so unfair to him, to call him, weeping beyond control to tell him I had cancer. How was he to deal with this? I sometimes wish I had done that differently, but maybe that was OK for Ron. He needed to have the time alone to deal with this. If you knew him, you would understand.

My second call was to my very best friend at that time, Kelly. I needed someone to take me to the doctor. I knew that I was in no shape to drive into West Health by myself and do this pre-op. Kelly, just like she did with everything else when I had cancer, dropped everything and came to my house to get me. I remember then picking up that Collie puppy named Callie and just hugging her, which is a strange thing, although I've always had a bond with animals. I'll probably never forget Callie either.

Then I went upstairs to take a shower. A couple other things that are real vivid to me happened that day. I remember standing in front of the shower taking all my clothes off to get in the shower and looking at my body and thinking, what is going on inside and how long has this been growing in me? What does my future hold? There were so many things I wanted out of life, and I stood there looking at myself and almost looking at my body like it was the enemy. I was thinking to myself, will I get to do all the things I want to do? Not even so much the things I want to do in terms of travel and the things I want to experience personally in my life, but the things I want to do for other people — nieces and nephews and being a part of their life for a long time, and in Ron's life, the life of friends and all that relationship stuff, then the things I want to experience in life.

I also remember thinking to myself, although this is in June, I don't know why I thought this or why it's so vivid to me, is that next Christmas, if I see Christmas, I'll put every decoration on my tree. I've always had a big tree, anywhere from 12 to 18 feet tall, and people have always given me lots of ornaments. I have hundreds, probably 300-400 ornaments. I'm sort of like everyone else. I get through the holidays. You get through Thanksgiving and you get through Christmas, and you get through to the New Year and you can't wait until summer. We're always getting through things. We're wishing our life away and need not to do that. We need to be here now. We need to experience Christmas and experience today. We need to open the window and smell that fresh manure that they're spreading on that field over there. We need to stop and smell the roses. We need to quit going so fast and so hard, where are we going? Be here now! We need to enjoy things today. At Christmas time we need to put up every village piece and put on every ornament. We need to go all out! We need to deck the halls! We just really need to live while we can live.

I remember going for my pre-op with Kelly and literally weeping all the way there, just crying. Crying my heart out. I had a lot of questions to ask the doctor. One of the questions I asked her because I knew I would be having a total hysterectomy was, "Will I grow whiskers?" I don't know why, but I've always thought women who have had a hysterectomy or been through their change or whatever get facial hair. She thought that was kind of funny, but I was quite concerned about having big old whiskers or a big old hair sticking out the mole on my nose or something like that. While I was there, I wept a little bit but kept my composure.

I had only met Dr. Maag once because of the whole series of events with that doctor that was sure I was too young for cancer. Dr. Maag was so warm and reassuring.

Now, the next difficult thing was that I was so afraid for Ron to come home, and I don't know why but I was afraid. It's so hard for Ron to feel and to cry, and I didn't want to put him through this. I didn't want to do cancer. Ron and I talked years before about either one of us ever getting cancer and that we would not do chemo; don't make or ask the other person to do chemo because we always thought that was the most nasty horrible thing that could happen to anyone in the world. So, I was so nervous for Ron to come home, and I remember watching him drive up the driveway, and I don't know why I was so afraid. He came in and we just hugged and held each other. He had gone to the company store at General Mills and bought me this t-shirt with a horse on it. It was Ron's way of telling me he was there for me.

Ed Dubois

The following article appeared in the **Dubious Distinctions Column** of the *Wright County Journal Press* the week after my surgery. The author of this column, Ed Dubois, has been a good friend, both personally and professionally, for more than a dozen years. Reading his column about me was, in many ways, like getting to read your own obituary before you die. I literally wept when I read Ed's column. It really meant a lot to me. And, it was a great way to "warn" everyone that I would be losing my hair.

Ed is a quiet, thoughtful man with a warm demeanor and an infectious smile. He and his family share a love for animals, which has brought us together on a number of occasions. Tasha Dubois (their smart little black dog) has spent some time at my house playing with the Heeter dogs when the Dubois family takes a vacation.

Thanks Ed, for your kind words and editorial support over the years.

Dubious Distinctions Column

There was a conspicuous absence at some of the Buffalo Days activities two weeks ago. When the indomitable one, Karla Heeter, was missing from the Pets in the Park event, Marlene Bresnahan explained that Karla was in the hospital. Marlene asked everyone to offer thoughts and prayers on Karla's behalf.

So full of energy and a love of life, Karla is not the sort of person you would expect to be slowed down by illness. A health problem would have to be pretty severe to send her to the hospital.

Many friends of Karla—and she has an abundance of them in the Buffalo area—must have been shocked when they learned a biopsy had revealed she had uterine and ovarian cancer and she had undergone surgery on Tuesday, June 10. She was released from the hospital on Saturday, June 14.

Instead of going home right away that day, Karla headed straight to the lure coursing (dog race) event at the local high school for "just a little bit." Two companions, long-legged Whippets which Karla has shown at Humane Society presentations, were competing.

"Staying at home ain't for me," Karla told me last week in her vivacious and colorful way. Although she underwent a hysterectomy and will soon begin chemotherapy, she said she feels confident she will be well again.

She mentioned having gone through some emotions over the past few weeks. Hearing that you have cancer can be overwhelming and can cause a person to get a little panicky, she said. Besides that, she said, due to her surgery, her hormones are "out of whack."

But she has been adjusting to this new "bridge I have to cross." Thinking ahead about the chemotherapy and losing her hair, she joked, "I'm looking for hats these days."

Karla is well known around here for her great gift of humor. Her "funshops" on the benefits of laughter have been a big hit with those who have attended.

Karla works for School District 877, where most of her time has been devoted to coordinating volunteers in the schools, promoting parental involvement and setting up school-community partnerships. But she is involved with so much more in the community. The Humane Society, the Community Health Foundation of Wright County, the new Safe Communities crash prevention program, a local saddle club, the local summer school Teen Team, senior citizen activities, and many charitable functions have all been touched by Karla's spirited involvement and infectious enthusiasm.

"I'm going to be all right," she is assuring her friends. She explained that medical science has come a long way in treating cancer. The outlook for patients is much better now than it was in the past.

Besides, you can't keep a person like Karla down for long. If anyone can face cancer and maintain a positive attitude, she can.

Last week, she was already talking about getting back to work.

"Staying home is not for me," she said. "I will get over this, and then it's back on the road again."

Keep Karla in mind when the Longest Day of Golf, the Relay for Life and the Cancer Golf Tournament take place this summer. Give generously and honor Karla for her courage and her uplifting, fortifying and encouraging spirit.

Dusty

Just a day or two after I returned home from the hospital following surgery, our good friends Karla and Noel and their two children, Ivy and Dusty, stopped in to see how I was doing. Karla's parents, Johnny and Diane, arrived at about the same time. I was perched in the recliner since that is where I felt most comfortable sitting.

We were visiting when I got this feeling that Dusty (about 9 or 10 years old at the time) wanted to say something. He would look at me and sort of cock his head sideways a little. The room got quiet and out of the blue he said to me, "Are you going to die?"

The room fell silent, and I mean you could have heard a pin drop. I'm quite sure that Dusty's mom and dad wished they were dead at that time. They could not believe what their son had just asked. It scared the life out of them.

Kids ask the things that we all wonder about. As adults we're looking for all the right words, and we don't know what to say to people. We don't know how to ask what the prognosis is, what are the doctors telling you, what are your chances for survival, can you beat this? Sometimes we need to ask people these things…but we don't. We're afraid to say, "What do you think, can you beat this or what's the prognosis?" and for Dusty to come out and say "Are you going to die?" was so honest and innocent and so necessary!

I guess I was sort of prepared for this. I knew that somewhere along the line someone, a child or an adult, would ask me if I was going to die and I needed to know what to say.

I know God gave me the words right then and there and I said, "You know, Dusty, I don't think I am. I think I'm going to live a long time. I'm going to work really hard at beating this, I want to live, and so you can know that I'm going to give it my best." I think that was so good for him. Dusty had lost someone in his life to cancer a few years earlier. All he knew at nine years old was that Sherry died. She had cancer and did not survive, so he needed to know if I was going to die.

Thanks Dusty for asking.

E – Energy and Enthusiasm

People know me as someone with a high level of energy and enthusiasm. I am type A, on the go, easily excitable, with what often seems like endless energy.

Chemotherapy robbed me of my energy. This was quite possibly the most disheartening and debilitating aspect of my cancer experience. I wanted to go, to be active, to stay involved, and sometimes I just couldn't. It was the one indicator, the most obvious characteristic to those around me that exemplified my fight for life.

I am thankful, every day, every hour, and every minute for my energy. You cannot show enthusiasm without energy, and I am proud of my genuine enthusiasm. It makes a difference in every aspect of my life. In all things, enthusiasm gets me where I'm going.

F – Feel

Another one of the good things to come from cancer is the ability it gives you to feel...to greater depths than ever before in life. I laugh harder, think deeper, smile more and cry easier...and that, as Martha Stewart would say, "is a good thing!"

Fun

Cancer helped me to see the value of fun. Life is short. Fun is important. We have to go for the gusto and pack a little fun in everyday.

So often we're saving fun for the weekend, the summer, our vacation or retirement. Don't save fun. Have fun today. There'll be more fun when the weekend comes, or vacation or whenever.

Figure out what your fun is, set some fun goals and make a plan for fun. If you don't, it may never happen.

I really believe that fun makes a difference in who we are, how we look and how healthy we are.

Have a little fun every day!

Faith Lutheran Church

In late February or early March of 1997 as my husband and I were driving from Monticello to Buffalo we passed yet another big new church under construction. As we discussed the cost of constructing this massive structure Ron said to me, "If you want to go to that little church out by Lake Maria State Park, I'll go with you." We went the next Sunday and have been happily involved there ever since.

We became members at another church in our early married years, but Ron didn't care to go. I felt uneasy about going alone, so I too quit going. The Lord knew we needed to be at Faith Lutheran Church. Just three months after we started going to this church, I was diagnosed with cancer. I cannot imagine facing cancer without a relationship with Jesus and a church family.

Many times during chemo it was all I could do, all the strength I could muster, to get to church, but I never missed…I needed to be there. Often times, I would weep. Many songs, scripture and prayers moved me to tears, as they do today. The music in my church is so meaningful. We are blessed to have a talented group of musicians who do such an awesome job with our music.

Pastor Tetlie's brother wrote the following piece that we sing at the end of our service. This song brings me such comfort.

> **Keep in mind God is with you**
>> **Keep in mind that you are free**
> **Keep in mind that God loves you**
>> **Even more than you believe**
>
> **Steadfast the love of God surrounds you**
>> **Ever more and in every way**
> **Never will God forsake or fail you**
>> **Steady flows the stream of grace**

Another song that appeared to be written specifically for what I was going through at the time is *For Those Tears I Died*. To this day, I weep every time we sing this song in church. It has so much meaning for me, especially because I am so often moved to tears when in church.

> **You said you'd come and share all my sorrows;**
>> **You said you'd be there for all my tomorrows.**
> **I came so close to sending you away,**
>> **But just as you promised you came there to stay,**
> **I just had to pray.**
>> **And Jesus said,**
>
> **"Come to the water, stand by my side.**
>> **I know you are thirsty, you won't be denied.**

I felt every tear drop when in darkness you cried,
    And I strove to remind you that for those tears I
died."

Your goodness so great I can't understand,
    And dear Lord, I know that all this was planned.
I know you're here now and always will be.
    Your love loosed my chains and in you I'm free.
But Jesus why me?
    And Jesus said,

"Come to the water, stand by my side.
    I know you are thirsty, you won't be denied.
I felt every tear drop when in darkness you cried,
    And I strove to remind you that for those tears I
died."

Jesus I give you my heart and my soul.
    I know now without God I'd never be whole.
Savior, you opened all the right doors,
    And I thank you and praise you from earth's
humble shores
    Take me I'm yours.
And Jesus said,

"Come to the water, stand by my side.
    I know you are thirsty, you won't be denied.
I felt every tear drop when in darkness you cried,
    And I strove to remind you that for those tears I
died."

Free Lunch

I worked in the Community Education Department at
District 877 Schools when I was diagnosed with cancer,
where it was commonplace for me to go out to lunch just
about every day. I either stepped out with a friend, a co-
worker, or a business associate. There was never a short-
age of lunch dates. Often, I turned away an invitation or
took a rain check.

    Now, having cancer, going through chemotherapy, and
losing your hair, had its benefits at lunchtime. You see, when

you're going through something of this magnitude, people want to help. They want to do anything and everything they can to let you know that they care, that they are pulling for you. Many times this comes in the form of "free lunch."

I cannot begin to count the number of times I was not allowed to pay for my lunch. I kind of grew to like this new benefit. I've learned that there is such a thing as "free lunch." But I don't recommend my method of getting there.

My thanks to all those lunch dates...all those who cared enough to feed me. Your friendship alone was enough to nourish me back to health!

G – Godparent

Being a Godparent, in my mind, has to be one of the highest honors bestowed on anyone. It implies that someone thinks you are worthy of caring for their child should the need arise, that your values and beliefs are of high standards and that you are loved.

In October of 1992, Ron and I were asked to be Godparents to our newborn niece Julia, daughter of Ron's nephew Scott and his wife Lisa. What an honor! We were surprised, overwhelmed and thoroughly delighted.

Just as I was about to begin chemotherapy treatments, my sister and her husband Terry asked if I, along with his father, would be Godparents for their new baby, Spencer. He was born on the day I had my endometrial biopsy. June 5, 1997. Again, I was surprised, overwhelmed and thoroughly delighted, although this time, I was a bit nervous about how I would feel on the Sunday of the baptism since I would have just had my first treatment.

Terry's dad was the best man in their wedding, and I was the maid of honor. What an honor that must have been for Terry's dad to be chosen by his son to be his best man. I, too, was honored to be in the wedding, but it is not common that a father serve his son as the best man. What a tribute to Bernard!

So, Shelley and Terry wanted the two of us to be Godparents. Ironically, we were both battling cancer and in chemotherapy at the time. I'll admit that it felt a bit odd to be a part of this ceremony, looking at Bernard and wondering how much time either of us would have with this precious little baby boy. Would we be a part of his life for years to come? I prayed that we would.

Bernard lost his life to colon cancer in August of 1997. He's in heaven watching over his grandson and Godchild, Spencer. I can only hope that Spencer continues to love his daddy, the way his daddy loved his daddy.

H – Humor

A sense of humor is one of the most important therapies available for fighting cancer. Humor helps us keep things in perspective. It lightens our load and it helps us to cope. Using humor makes it easier for those around us to deal with the entire cancer experience. It opens the door to conversation and helps us to connect. After all, laughter is the shortest distance between two people.

Humor and laughter are important survival tools!

Hats

Hats were a mainstay in my wardrobe for almost eight months. I had casual hats, dressy hats, funny hats, ugly hats, cute hats, you name it, and I had it. People from all aspects of my life showered me with hats. I can actually say that I miss wearing hats now; it was fun to accessorize with hats. Many people told me that they missed my hats after my hair came back. They became a part of my personality. Not everyone can wear hats, but since I have a round face, I wear hats well.

A special thanks to all those who gave me hats. The gift of a hat when you've lost your hair is not unlike giving mittens to the homeless in Minnesota. Like Campbell's soup, "It warms you heart and soul."

Heyerdahl

Following my surgery in the hospital I got a phone call from a teacher that worked in the same building that I did. We had a number of interactions in the school, visited in the hall periodically, but were not particularly close, not friends outside of the confines of the school day.

This teacher, Jan Heyerdahl, called the day after my surgery. I was a bit down and maybe even somewhat weepy. We visited for a while about my surgery when she began to tell me how God had a plan for me. That was hard for me to see or understand at that time, but from that day forward, Jan and I had a connection, a faith connection.

She continued to support me and to nurture my faith through my treatments. A few months later, I called her up and asked her, as an English Teacher, to help me narrate a coloring book about cancer prevention and early detection for the children of Wright County. She was phenomenal at this task. Writing in rhyme comes naturally to her. Not only was she good at writing but also she really seemed to be connected with the concepts and ideas I wanted to portray to the kids. We narrated this coloring book in literally minutes.

About six months after the coloring book narration, Jan and I had lunch together and she began telling me about this breast lump that she had and as time passed she'd continue to have mammograms and be asked to "wait and see." I hounded her about getting a second opinion and as it is so typical with Jan, she "had a peace about this." She put her faith in God and let Him guide her decisions.

Jan was diagnosed with breast cancer that spring, and her story lies ahead. She has been an inspiration to me. Her faith is as solid as a rock, and her friendship has been a blessing. I can only hope that I have been as helpful to Jan on her cancer journey as she was to me on mine.

I am honored to share my story on the same pages as Jan. She has been so instrumental in helping me grow in my faith. The process of putting our journey in print has been powerful, therapeutic, healing, and humbling.

I love you, Girlfriend!

I – Inspiration

To be told that you are an inspiration to someone is the highest compliment one can pay you. Many times through my battle with cancer people told me that I was an inspiration to them. They would say that they marveled at my positive attitude, the way I faced the sometimes-difficult treatment and my constant desire to maintain my involvement with the outside world.

It's humbling to think that "I" could inspire others. Certainly, I had to play the hand that was dealt me and I had a choice. I could play it with hope, humor and zest, or I could wallow in self-pity, negativity and woe. I chose to live everyday to the fullest. To this day, I continue to live as though it were my last day!

To those who offered this ultimate compliment, I thank you...and know that my strength comes from the Lord.

J – Jeannie Fobbe

People are so critical to the cancer experience! From diagnosis day, through surgery and chemo, people came to the call for me. Whether it was a family member, someone from my church, a friend, a neighbor or a co-worker, people really were my strength and my salvation. Knowing others cared and were pulling for me made all the difference in the world.

Often times in my presentations I say that I wish everyone in the room could experience cancer because it changes your life. You realize what's important, what's most valuable in life. It's people and relationships! When it's all said and done, and we draw our last breath, it's not going to matter if we're driving a Lexus or a Lincoln, a Honda or a Chevy. It won't matter if we live in the biggest, most beautiful house in the new development in town or if we're in a modest apartment. When we draw that last breath, what really matters, is the difference we make in the lives of people.

Many people touched my life during my cancer experience. One person who was there for me 200% was my dear friend, Jeannie Fobbe. She called; she stopped over; she sent cards and she sent cards and she sent cards. I don't think a day went by from diagnosis day through my last chemo treatment that I did not open the mailbox and know that Jeannie was thinking about me, supporting me and was there for me! Everyday, there was a card, a note or a little something from Jeannie. (Confetti included!)

Jeannie knows how to make people feel good and has a marvelous ability to nurture relationships. She genuinely cares about people. Jeannie cares little about material things and much about family and friends. She exudes warmth! Everybody loves Jeannie. We all need a Jeannie Fobbe in our lives! It's the "Jeannies" that make the world a better place.

Jamie

All my life it's been important to me to make a difference. Since my cancer experience it is a passion, a burning desire. Hardly a day goes by when I don't ask myself what contribution I have made. Have I made a difference in someone's day...in his or her life? I have the opportunity to do that often with my work on the Wright Cancer Hotline. Being a mentor through the United for Youth Sidekicks Mentor Program affords me that same opportunity to make a difference as well.

In the fall of 1999, I was matched with a very special little girl named Jamie, a beautiful blonde fourth grader with a smile that warms the entire room. Our time together has been so rewarding. I often wonder who is benefiting more from our time together...she or I?

Mentoring is such a simple thing to do and so rewarding. Yet, so few people will take the time and make the commitment. I am convinced that if every adult would get involved in the life of one child, the world would be a different place. Every child needs to know that they have an adult who cares about them, someone they can trust.

We should all step back at some point in our lives and ask ourselves, "How do I want to be remembered? What will people say when they reminisce about me? What contribution have I made to my family, community, church, mankind, etc.?" And then, live accordingly!

Thanks Jamie, for being a part of my life. I can only hope our friendship is as important to you as it is to me.

K – Kelly

I imagine anyone who has been through the cancer experience would tell you that they had one special person, that good friend, who really helped them get through the entire ordeal. They had someone who supported them, helped them through difficult days, did special favors, sort of just always knew what to do, what to say, how to help.

That person for me was my friend Kelly. She took me to pre-op, went with me for surgery, chored my horses when I was in the hospital, held my spot on our equestrian drill team, put hay up in my barn, and anything else I needed. She was there for me physically and emotionally. I will be forever grateful to Kelly for her unending support and friendship through this life-changing event.

Koosh Kash

In the midst of my cancer treatments, I took a business trip to Washington, DC with my boss, Chuck, an Advisory Council Member, Idella, and one of our school partners and good friend, Sonja.

When Sonja and I arrived in DC, we flagged a taxi. We instructed the driver to take us to the Embassy Suites. When the driver pulled up at the wrong Embassy, he had words with another taxi driver, neither of them speaking English. After this brief exchange, the other driver took a look at the two of us and brusquely said, "Foo Foo" to our driver and we sped off. Sonja asked him what this meant and he sheepishly said, "It is a type of food in my country." We were sure this wasn't really true and have endearingly greeted each other with these words ever since.

Earlier, on a conference call with the team that we were training with at this focused learning series, we over-heard one of our team leaders talk about a colleague whose last name sounds like Koosh Kash. Thinking this is a really cool name; this too, has stuck with us. Now, we affectionately call each other Foo Foo or Koosh Kash.

I had finished three or four treatments when we went to DC, so I was sportin' a hat. Our group was required to make a presentation. Since we were a creative team, we wrote a song to introduce our project. And, because I had to wear a hat, the rest of the team honored me and also wore hats for our presentation.

Sonja works at the Buffalo Hospital and was one of our strongest school partners. Our jobs paralleled a great deal, and we were involved in a number of community-wide projects and initiatives at the time of my cancer diagnosis. Through our professional association, we became good friends.

I love spending time with Sonja. I love being around positive people who like to have fun! And, that's my Koosh Kash!

L – Loneliness

Probably the single most difficult aspect of the entire cancer experience for me was loneliness. While many people get their strength from time alone, my strength comes from people. I love people. I love to be with people. Time alone for me is like punishment.

There is a different kind of loneliness that comes from illness or personal tragedy. The feeling that no matter how many cards, letters, phone calls, prayers, visits and flowers you may receive, the fact remains that it is "I" that is experiencing this disease and only "I."

Since my need for people was so strong, I continued to work through my treatments. When I look back, it scares me to think that I went to work, at a school, nonetheless, even when my blood counts were dangerously low. I didn't want to stay home. Again, this was like punishment for me to have to stay away from people. I literally risked my life because I didn't want to stay home and be alone.

My treatments took place on a Monday and Tuesday every three weeks and then I would be at home, usually in bed, for the next three or four days. I wasn't necessarily sick on those days, but I was TIRED. You can't know tired unless you've known the kind of tired that chemotherapy gives you. And even though I would be in bed and sleeping most of the time, it was lonely. I would wake up and roll over and know everybody was at work and the world was going on out there. Things were happening all over the world without me. There were cars passing my house, people laughing over a glass of wine at lunch, others accomplishing great things in their work place, and camaraderie in my office that was happening without me. It's just such an alone feeling.

It's important to me that people know about and remember how important it is to seek out people who are experiencing difficult times in their lives. We need to be there for people when they need us most. Often this means putting others before ourselves. It makes all the difference in the world when you know people care.

M – Dr. Maag

Dr. Maag, my Ob-Gyn has made a difference in my life.

Her warmth, positive reassurance and extensive know-ledge have been key to my survival. She is indeed a very competent, thorough, caring physician. Unlike other doc-tors I've met, she sits down and listens, not with her arm full of charts and one hand on the doorknob, but right in front of you, with her undivided attention. She listens.

The first time I met her, I knew that we would have a lasting relationship. She seemed human, like she was con-cerned about my symptoms and that we would get to the bottom of this. After I had been doctoring somewhere else for several months with these same symptoms, Dr. Maag's determination was reassuring to me.

One of the most important things Dr. Maag did for me was to act! Yes, to take action, to find out what was the cause for my symptoms. She was prompt in getting my results to me and equally as prompt in getting me in for surgery. All this sounds so simple, like, isn't that the way it should be? Yes, it should, but how many times do people have a biopsy, a CT scan or MRI and wait days, or even weeks for a response? Waiting and wondering is often more difficult than the diagnosis itself.

What a comfort it was to have Dr. Maag there when my mother experienced cancer just eight months after I was diagnosed. I knew she would be just as kind, caring, thor-ough and prompt with my mom. And, she delivered my newest nephew, Tyler, just a couple months ago. She truly is like family.

Another great thing about Dr. Maag is that I feel like she is genuinely excited to see me when I go in for check ups. I feel like she really cares and is concerned about my continued good health.

I'm sure glad I found Dr. Maag.

Massage

During all six of my chemotherapy treatments, my dear friend Lori would come to the hospital and spend the evening with me. Ron would leave in the late afternoon,

I'd take a nap or do some reading and Lori would show up at suppertime. I thoroughly enjoyed our time together, just talking "girl talk," and I absolutely loved her foot massages. Lori gave me a foot massage during every single treatment. She'd use that good smelling hospital lotion, and massage my feet for what seemed like hours. What a kind, nurturing act of friendship. Thanks Lori, for being there and for your friendship.

Many times in the week after my treatment, I would schedule a full-body massage with one of my massage therapist friends, Sue or Jeannie. Massage is so healing, it releases the toxins in your body, helps you to relax, and just plain makes you feel alive and well. Thanks, Sue and Jeannie, for sharing your time and talents to help me get through chemo.

N – Numb Feet and Nausea

Two very annoying, yet short-lived aspects of my treatment for cancer were numb feet and nausea. Both are gone and nearly forgotten, yet in the midst of undergoing the chemotherapy (Taxol and Cysplatin) that I needed to survive, they were both troublesome side effects.

It's imperative that we keep things in perspective and stay positive, even about the difficult battles we encounter. At the time, numb feet and nausea seemed insurmountable; in retrospect, they were a pretty minor price to pay for life.

O – Ovarian Cancer

Gilda's Disease...how ironic that I would get "Gilda's Disease." I am someone who thinks that Gilda Radner was one of the greatest comedians in my lifetime. She is the only person I had ever heard of, or known, who got ovarian cancer. I remember hearing about Gilda's death at such a very young age from ovarian cancer. I had read her book called *It's Always Something* and remember thinking how scary and helpless it must have been to battle such a hopeless disease. And now, I too, could lose my life in the same way Gilda had.

Ovarian cancer is called the silent killer. Because it is so difficult to diagnose, by the time it is detected, it is usually in the late stages and cannot be cured.

I remember waking up from the anesthesia in my hospital room and hearing my husband tell others in the room and on the phone that surgery had revealed not only uterine cancer but ovarian cancer as well. And in that groggy state, I silently wept, tears falling past my temple, onto my pillow, knowing that this was much more serious than we had ever imagined.

Indeed I would learn that both of my cancers were STAGE 1, both encapsulated! My cancer was caught early. Yet, the cytology wash revealed cancer cells in the peritoneal fluids in the pelvic and abdominal area. I would need chemotherapy as "an insurance policy," to be sure no other cells would continue to grow.

The Lord has blessed me. I survived! I get to tell the story, to help others, to live and love and serve the Lord! My story would not end like Gilda's.

Optimism

I am an optimist to a fault. I live by the saying, "If you think you can, you can...and if you think you can't, you're right!" So often, people are given a diagnosis of cancer and decide that they cannot survive, and indeed, they do not.

In all aspects of life, we can choose success or failure. It's a decision we make at work, at home, in relationships and with all other challenges in life. I've heard it said, "Life is 10% what you make it and 90% how you take it." And so it is with each of us, it's up to us to make the best of what life brings our way.

P – Prayers

"Sometimes PRAYER is the only gift we can give one another."

So many people prayed for me. Early on, I was uncomfortable when someone told me that they would pray for me. I often wanted to say, "Oh, you don't need to do that! Don't use up your prayers on me." I felt guilty that they were spending their prayers on me. More importantly, I thought it meant that I was weak or needy.

I now know the power of prayer. I was indeed, weak and needy. I needed prayers. Truly, I believe that prayers got me through this most difficult time in my life.

Time and time again someone would call and say, "I heard about your cancer through my prayer chain." People of all faiths were praying for me. People near and far. People that I didn't even know had a relationship with the Lord were praying for me. How often I was surprised by someone's gesture of prayer.

I am so grateful to have so many people in my life who know the power of prayer! Let ME now offer praise!

Pam Link

One Sunday after my third or fourth chemo, I noticed a bouquet of red roses on the altar at church. Someone had offered roses in honor or in memory of a loved one.

After the service, Pam Link, one of our talented musicians said, "Somebody should take these roses home. They'll never keep until next Sunday." She walked up to the altar, took the bouquet in her hands and said, "Here, Karla, you take these. You deserve a bouquet of roses!" There I stood, hairless, weak from chemo, and nearly moved to tears. I don't know why I was so touched by this simple gesture on that day, but I do know that I cried all the way home...with that bouquet of roses on my lap.

It just goes to show you that we never know how we

will touch people with our random acts of kindness or a simple gesture like this. As a newcomer to Faith, I had watched Pam from the pews and thought she was a pretty wonderful person. I will never forget the roses Pam gave me on that Sunday at church.

Q – Quit...Don't Quit

In my darkest days, following my most difficult chemotherapy treatment (number four), I received these Hallmark words of encouragement from my friend Sue Sopkin. It's amazing how the Lord works through people. As I seriously contemplated not finishing my final two treatments, this verse helped put things in perspective for me. I would continue with my treatments...for life!

Don't Quit...

When things go wrong, as they sometimes will,
　　When the road you're trudging
Seems all uphill,
　　When the funds are low
And the debts are high,
　　And you want to smile
But you have to sigh,
　　When care is pressing you
Down a bit,
　　Rest if you must
But don't you quit.
　　Life is queer with its twists and turns,
As every one of us sometimes learns,
　　And many a failure turns about,
When you might have won
　　Had you stuck it out.
Don't give up, though the pace seems slow—
　　You may succeed with another blow.
Success is failure turned inside out—
　　The silver tint of the clouds of doubt.
And you never can tell
　　How close you are;
It may be near when it seems so far.

So stick to the fight
When you're hardest hit—
It's when things seem worst
That you must not quit.

R – Ron...my husband and my best friend

They say that a cancer diagnosis, or any other life changing event that we may experience will "make or break" a marriage. The relationship will never be the same. It is so true.

Cancer brought us closer, gave us an ability to communicate in a way we had not been able to in the past. It helped us to realize how important we are to each other, how we must not miss any opportunity to tell each other how we feel, how appreciative we are to have this time together. To realize that we must LIVE! Now, today...with gusto! Do the things we have always dreamed of. Make plans, set goals, and follow our dreams.

My husband Ron is shy. He is also one of those men who shows very little emotion. He's not too excitable, has rarely ever been seen with a tear on his cheek and isn't much of a communicator, especially on a feeling level. But, you will know when he is there for you. He is faithful and diligent to his commitments in life!

About three weeks after my surgery, which would have been about two weeks before my chemo treatments were to begin, a number of people had asked how Ron was doing with all this. Because he is so shy and rarely talks about how he feels, I'm sure people were concerned. After telling people, "Oh, he's just fine. You know Ron, he doesn't say too much." I asked him. I said, "You know, Ron, everyone's asking me how you're doing. I keep telling them you seem to be handling this all quite well, but how are you doing?" He looked at me with a very serious, yet somewhat uncertain look on his face and said, "I'll be just fine as long as you don't die on me."

S – *South Dakota*

One of my life dreams came true shortly after I was diagnosed with cancer. The day after my second chemotherapy treatment we left, with nine other families, to ride our horses in the Black Hills of South Dakota.

It was a long, hot trip, taking nearly 16 hours to reach our destination. I was quite sick on the drive, having to lie down almost all the way there. But, I wasn't going to miss this trip for anything, not even cancer. In all honesty, I went on this trip, sort of thinking in the back of my mind, that it quite possibly would be my last trip.

Originally, we had planned to stay in a tent. Others in our group had reserved the few cabins offered at the resort, so we were going to sleep outside. Fortunately, my friend Kelly suggested that we share their cabin with them. What a Godsend! I would not have been able to survive that trip, with the temperatures dipping into the 30's and 40's in the night. Again, Kelly was there for me!

I was pretty nervous about our first trail ride, not sure if I was strong enough to endure the ride in the hills, and if not, how would I get back to camp? More than two dozen of us saddled our horses and prepared to head out on the trail. Now, with this many people getting ready to ride, we often end up waiting for 15 – 30 minutes for the whole crew to ride out. I sat on my horse in the hot sun for about 10 minutes before I realized that I should get off before I fall off. I was light headed and about to faint.

I stepped down off my horse and lay in the cool grass under the shade of a tree. Fighting tears, I encouraged the group to go on without me. My husband Ron stayed with me and as the group rode off into the hills; I wept. This was one of those times when I felt so lonely that it hurt.

Ron and I went up to the cabin where I sat for 15-20 minutes and regrouped. I was so determined to ride. Once I felt a bit better, we set out on what literally turned out to be the ride of a lifetime. We took a trail that circled a magnificent lake with some absolutely breath-taking views, just the two of us. The truth is, we kind of got lost, took a different trail than we thought we were on and were gone for more than four hours.

Ron was so patient, so concerned, so supportive and so loving on that ride. God knew we needed that time together, to be with each other and see His beauty!

The rest of the week in South Dakota was filled with gorgeous rides, good friends and a number of other rich experiences. I'm so thankful that I got to fulfill this dream.

Smoke

I was standing out by the buses one day as students were departing at the end of the school day. I was wearing a hat, but it was easy to see that I had no hair. One little boy looked up at me curiously. I could tell he was wondering about my lack of hair. I asked him if he wanted to see my baldhead to which he enthusiastically replied, "yah." He said, "You have cancer, don't you?" I said, "Yes I do." He instantly blurted out, "You smoke, don't you?" I said, "No I don't." To which he insisted, "You do, too!" When I again denied that I smoke, he said, "Then why do you have cancer if you don't smoke?"

I'd say we've done an excellent job educating young people about the perils of smoking. Why then, are so many young people smoking today?

T – Tata Head

During my second chemotherapy treatment I lost almost all of my hair. While in the hospital for that treatment, my hair was everywhere, on the bed, the floor, in the bathroom...everywhere. It came out in clumps. I could literally run my hands through my hair and gather clumps of hair between my fingers.

When I got home from that second treatment, I looked

as though I was diseased, with areas of my head totally bald and a few spots where I had a clump of hair left. I needed to take control of the situation and remove the rest of my hair. I was leaving in just two days for a trip I had looked forward to for a lifetime – our trip to South Dakota to ride our horses in the Black Hills.

I called my good friend and hairdresser Lisa and asked if she would come to my house and shave my head. She arrived with clippers, scissors and Bic razors. The clipper job looked a bit strange, so she used the Bic razor and shaved my head. We're talking Kojak! No hair—totally bald! It was early August, and I was quite tan. My scalp was white, and I mean white. I looked like an alien, or a Saturday Night Live Conehead without the cone. It was shocking.

Knowing that I wanted to "break the ice" with a few friends before we left for our trip to South Dakota, I went to my friend Kelly's house. I put a baseball cap on, but you could still see my virgin white scalp at my temples and on the back of my neck. When I arrived, Kelly's three-year-old son, Tommy, looked at me with curiosity and asked me to take off my hat. (We had prepared him prior to this...telling him that the medicine I had to take for cancer would make my hair fall out.) His eyes got big and he grinned and said, "Kar, you look like a Tata head." (Mr. Potato head) Tommy was one of the first to see me without hair and from that day forward, many called me "Tata Head"

Toys

I was the recipient of a number of toys throughout my hospital stays and treatment period. One of my favorite toys was a Tickle Me Elmo doll from my good friend Jeannie. It made me laugh.

Another of my favorite toys was a cultivator from Tommy, the little boy who gave me the name Tata Head. He had been hospitalized for a brief overnight stay shortly before I went in for my surgery. During that hospital-ization, he was given a little cultivator that he actually slept with on that night. He convinced his mommy that Karla Heeter, too, needed a cultivator while in the hospital. I still have that precious gift in its original box.

When we grow up, we often forget the importance of play. Spending time with toys, giving toys and playing with them helps us to remember the value of play. We need to spend time in play, to recognize our playful hearts.

U – Utterberg

Having experienced symptoms for more than eight months and getting nowhere with the doctor I had been seeing for several months, I took the advice of my good friend and hair dresser Lisa Utterberg to see her Ob-Gyn. She had experienced similar problems and had total con-fidence in Dr. Linda Maag. Not only was she confident with her medical expertise, she was extremely pleased with her "bedside manner." She was convinced that I would really like Dr. Maag.

Knowing that seeing a different doctor would require switching providers through my husband's insurance car-rier at work, I reluctantly went through the motions, got the paper work in order and made my appointment to see this new "lady doctor." I had always had a "man doctor," except for the "lady doctor" who thought I was "too young for cancer" and didn't take me seriously enough to diag-nose this cancer that was growing inside me.

So, I made my appointment with Dr. Maag and the rest is history! Lisa's advice to see her doctor saved my life. And in the process, she lost my business for the next 8 – 10 months because I had no hair.

In addition to leading me to this wonderful new doctor, Lisa helped me learn about wigs, brought food to my house, sent cards and called on a regular basis. She, like so many others, stood by me through the whole cancer experience.

I will always see Lisa as my lifesaver! She encouraged me to see her doctor and I am alive! Thanks Lisa!

V – Victory

I survived! I beat cancer! What a Victory!
- **H**umor
- **A**ttitude
- **P**eople
- **P**rayer
- **Y**es, I'm Happy!

Vita Mix

It amazes me that we have to get a kick in the seat of the pants to move us to a healthy lifestyle. It also amazes me how quickly we forget the urgency of that healthy lifestyle and fall back into old habits.

Before I started chemotherapy, my husband bought a Vita-Mix machine. We mixed fruits and veggies with the skins to get all the nutrients we could. I even bought all organic fruits and vegetables. I no longer use my Vita-Mix machine for fruit and veggie shakes, but it sure makes a mean Mudslide.

In addition to my healthy drinks, I also saw an alternative doctor during chemotherapy and took a number of supplements to help me get through the treatments. I really do think that eating healthy and taking my supplements made a big difference in my strength and stamina during chemo.

Now, if I could just stay committed to these healthy habits.

W – Water

As I was about to leave the hospital after my surgery, my oncologist stopped in for some final words on my treatment plan. I got dressed and said to her, "Well, now what? How do I live? Is there anything I should do differently?

Should I change my eating habits? How should I live?" She looked at me and said, "The first thing I'd do is get rid of that diet pop, if you must drink pop, drink regular pop, not diet. It's full of chemicals and carcinogens. Otherwise, just carry on, live as you have in the past."

And, that is the one major change I have made in my life. I drink lots and lots of water. Only on occasion, do I drink pop.

Mary Ellen Wells

Until we experience a life-changing event like cancer, we often do not see what people are really made of. When the going gets tough, we then see who comes to the call, who's really there for us and who steps up to the plate to see you through the difficult times.

One of the first people to call me on diagnosis day, as the news about my cancer spread like wild fire, was a woman who I had primarily known as a professional associate, but soon to be a very dear friend. Mary Ellen Wells, President of the Buffalo Hospital and fellow member of the Community Health Foundation Board of Directors was sitting on the interview committee for the Foundation Executive Director position that I was to interview for later that day.

I picked up the phone, obviously shaken and distraught, in tears and afraid, and Mary Ellen said, "Karla, it's Mary Ellen, I heard about your diagnosis. Tell me, what can I do? I'll go to surgery with you; I can meet you there. I know lots of people at Abbott, I'll be sure you get the best care available. I want to help—just tell me what I can do. If you don't want or need me to be involved, just say so, I'm OK with that, but I want to help."

I will never forget Mary Ellen's call. The confidence in her voice, her genuine desire to help, her commitment to see me through this difficult time will never be forgotten.

I took Mary Ellen up on her offer. She met us at the

door at the hospital on that uncertain day and was there with my husband Ron, my friend Kelly, and my Pastor Jim as I was prepared for surgery. We laughed, we cried and we prayed. What an awesome support team.

Thanks Mary Ellen, from the bottom of my heart!

Women of Excellence

As a cancer survivor, I often find myself thinking about and being thankful for so many of the events and happenings in my life. It might be something as simple as a ride in the park on my horse, sitting on the sofa with one of my dogs or just "being with" my husband Ron. Or, it may be something as significant as helping someone on the Wright Cancer Hotline, reaching someone through one of my speaking engagements or receiving one of the Monticello Women of Excellence awards.

I am "a Woman of Excellence!" I was nominated and chosen to receive one of the Monticello Women of Excellence Awards in April of 2000. The nomination itself is a great honor, to be chosen as a recipient is overwhelming. That someone believed I was worthy of this recognition is humbling. Even more humbling was the show of support from members of my church at the Awards Banquet.

I got to live to be a Woman of Excellence. Kim Garberich, your nomination touched my heart. Thanks for thinking I'm worthy!

X – Humor Xchange

Since the early 90's I've been doing public speaking. Most people would rather die than speak in front of people. Not me… I love an audience! Any day I get out of bed, and get to speak to an audience, is a great day.

I was employed in the school system as the Community Partnership Facilitator. I worked with parents, students, volunteers, business partners and all levels of school staff. It was a great job with a lot of a variety and tons of people stuff, just what I like. Although I liked the safety and security of having an employer, with benefits, co-workers, and all that comes with a traditional job, I decided that I wanted to follow my passion. I was passionate about speaking. It was time to take that big leap and start my own business. After much thought and consideration, I named my new business *Humor Xchange.*

I had dabbled in the speaking business for a number of years and just before my cancer diagnosis had actually gotten quite busy at it. Chemotherapy mandated that I cancel all of my engagements for about six months. Since most of my business comes from those who have heard me, I wasn't sure if I'd be able to rekindle my speaking business after chemo. I literally had to call everybody on my calendar to tell them I had been diagnosed with cancer and would be undergoing chemo and wouldn't know how I would be feeling, so I had to relinquish many jobs.

A week after my final chemo I had a speaking engagement at Delano. I couldn't cancel. I needed to get back in the swing of my speaking to feel normal again. I even remember what I wore to this presentation. I was so weak, but the speaking engagement went so well.

The rewards from speaking are so abundant. I really feel like I have an opportunity to touch people, to affect lives, and to make a difference. The following e-mail message that I received after one of my presentations illustrates that reward.

This is why I speak!

Hi Karla,

I was at your presentation this past Wednesday in St. Cloud—it was for the Lifeline people. You gave me a coloring book . . . remember me, I work at North Memorial?

After the drive up there on Wednesday I could

barely turn my head because my neck was so stiff—you helped that!

I must share with you the following:

Though I generally like most people I have found over the past three years that there are some that when I see them—don't even have to talk with them—I just know they are full of spirit. That special spirit that one can only acquire when they have gone though great difficulty. I instinctly feel a bond with this person—even if I never speak with them— it is something in their eyes.

On 5/96 I went in for routine surgery on my thyroid—a cyst, no big deal—and when I woke up I was told it was more, it was cancer . . . that big CCCCC. Well, having worked with hospice (Monticello-Big Lake Hospice office) to me cancer equaled death. The saga continued with a surgeon that did not remove the thyroid and I had to go in for surgery again—but had to wait for at least six months! Anyway that summer I was convinced that all this meant that I was going to die and so I must prepare my two children (Jen/15 and John/14) my husband would be fine, but my children, especially my John. He and I were two of a kind—sort of scary!!!

Jen and my husband really refused to look at my feelings or the possibilities—after all this was a "good" kind of cancer to have. Oh, I must back up, throughout my life I have always had an ability to "sense" things. So, I had this sense and I KNEW that there was going to be a death.

One beautiful day my son and I went out fishing up on Pelican Lake—had a great time, picnic in the boat—no fish so why not eat! As we crossed the lake I asked him what he thought about God and heaven—as he could always see through me, he knew what I was getting at. So I backed off.

Then a few weeks later the most beautiful Monarch butterfly was on a flower—it just stayed there and I call him and his buddy down to see this and it still didn't move, just ate from that flower. I felt such a power from this little butterfly—I told the boys that what we were watching was creation/universe/God, you name it, in action and to never forget this moment—this was a moment of great meaning.

Before we left for the cities the lake was like glass—it was Labor Day Weekend and fabulous. John and I always skied together (water skiing was a passion of mine since age 7 and I too like the sound/feel of "hitting it" in the boat!) John refused—that was odd. We loaded up the car and as we pulled out I had a wave and I looked at my husband and said—it will never be the same again.

I was scheduled for my second surgery (new doc and new hospital) on 10/20 something. As the time approached I even cleaned out the junk drawer—there again was this sense—I must have it ready, if I die people can't know what a closet slob I was!!!

On October 15, at 6:38 p.m. I came upon an accident on 169 in Elk River—that is where we used to live. I looked over and saw John's friends all screaming and I didn't see John. I knew. As I crossed over the lanes of traffic I saw my beautiful spirited boy just lying there. He looked so peaceful and I knew that no matter what they did he would not be coming home that night. My precious gift had been taken from me.

I cancelled the surgery for the next week but had to have it. So about three weeks later I went in— fully convinced that God had taken my love because he could not have survived my death. Looking back on the scene, that poor anesthesiologist, he asked me if I was sure I wanted to do this. I think he was afraid I would will myself to death and he would be responsible!!! (Humor in healthcare!)

But I lived—dahhhh! In recovery I was surrounded by John and his angel friends—even the PACU nurse thought it was odd that I was so peaceful and needed no morphine or anything. What a peaceful experience that was. This was the first of many "signs" that have helped me to survive.

Now you may think . . . who is this nut case and why is she opening her heart to me. I must say, for the private person I am, this is an odd one. The only thing I can think of is you touched me. Maybe it is one survivor seeing another survivor. Again, it was the eyes. Have you ever felt that with people? (This is the point where you validate that I am not a NUT!) Survivors have a special gleam—depth, something in their eyes.

I have had to learn to laugh again—I work at it—my husband thinks I am a bit off because each night I must see one of the re-runs of Third Rock—and I laugh—even when I am all alone.

So perhaps I had to tell you all this because what you do for a living is what helped me get through the darkest days one can imagine. Or perhaps if you got me one step closer to saying that I am a cancer survivor—Ohhhh, just writing it makes me look over my shoulder for another boulder!

I have passed on the information on the upcoming workshop—I dont' know if I can attend it—why do I still have fear from this cancer!?

Anyway Ms. Karla Heeter . . . I think you are a terrific speaker and I want you to remember me on those days that you sometimes are wondering what it is all about (we all have those days from time to time). You make a difference—your gift helped another along this journey we call life.

Thank you for listening and thank you for being YOU!

Most sincerely/fondly,
Linda

P.S. That coloring book—I used to LOVE coloring with my kids. When I get around to it I will color you the one in the book with the butterfly sitting on the rose . . . now what are the chances that would be in the book you gave to me . . . powerful isn't it?!!!!!

Y – Yesterday is Gone

All too often we spend too much time in yesterday. We worry and fret about things that have already happened, things we can do nothing about. Yesterday is gone, we must live for today. Having cancer helped me to put worry into perspective and realize how important it is to move forward and make the most of TODAY!

The following little reading often serves as a reminder for me that worry is a waste of precious time.

Worry Table

Stress management experts say that 2% of the average person's worrying is spent on things that might be helped or somehow improved by worrying. The other 98% is spent (or wasted) as follows:

40% on things that never happen
35% on things that can't be changed
15% on things that turn out better than expected
8% on useless, petty worries

An obvious (though hard to abide by) conclusion: **consciously refuse to worry about anything unless you have good reason to believe that worrying about it can actually do some good.**

Z – Zest for Life

Zest for Life is about appreciating our surroundings; being thankful for what we have; counting our blessings. So many people have great health, wealth, family and friends, loved ones, church, jobs, and all kinds of "stuff," yet they don't have a zest for life.

I wonder sometimes if it's that they don't have a relationship with the Lord that keeps them from appreciating what they have. And I think many times if we were to really look at lives that lack zest, that is exactly what's missing. To have zest for life, you have to have a relationship with the Lord. Knowing that you are free, that you are loved and that with God, all things are possible, in and of itself, creates a zest for life. He is the Activity Director; He is the Ultimate Planner and Organizer. Believing in Him will set you free to live without fear.

> **Let him have all your worries and cares, for He is always thinking about you and watching everything that concerns you.**
>
> *1 Peter 5:7*

> **Don't worry about anything; instead, pray about everything; tell God your needs and don't forget to thank Him for his answers. If you do this you will experience God's peace, which is far more wonderful that the human mind can understand. His peace will keep your thoughts and hearts quiet and at rest as you trust in Christ Jesus.**
>
> *Philippians 4:6, 7*

Conclusion

In conclusion of my LMNOP writings, I would like to share an insightful quote from Joanna Bull's forward in M. Steven Piver and Gene Wilder's book *Gilda's Disease*. Her words about Gene Wilder parallel my thoughts, feelings and purpose for this book. To bring meaning to this entire cancer experience and to appreciate the splendor of life are the essence of our stories.

> "Gene Wilder is here, sharing the too common saga of Mr. and Mrs. Gene Wilder's search for and explanation of Gilda's symptoms, a search that finally led to ovarian cancer—which had, tragically, been there all along. Gene Wilder's oversized heart is so constituted that he must always search further, for the meaning that's hidden in confusion. He found it in "Gilda's great gift" to him and to us. Gene's advice for husbands and significant others can be extended to all human beings who are reminded through illness that we are mortal and *it is that very fact* that gives every minute of our living its preciousness."

Jan's Story

My journey began when I detected a change in my left breast during a breast self-exam. It was not a pea or a marble; it was a thickening, a firmness on the outer edge of my breast. Four mammograms revealed nothing. Two ultrasounds followed, and the radiologist said I was fine! Unsatisfied with the lack of explanation for the change in my breast, I met with my gynecologist, who referred me on to a surgeon, who offered to "watch it a month, do another mammogram, or try a needle biopsy." Wanting expediency, I requested the needle biopsy. The results came back "suspicious," so, an incision biopsy was performed. Finally the results were conclusive: lobular carcinoma.

Less than 15% of breast cancers are lobular carcinomas. They are difficult to detect and have a more notorious reputation for recurring in the other breast. Eight days after diagnosis I underwent a bilateral mastectomy with a TRAM flap. (Reconstruction was made with a Transverse Rectus Abdominus Myocutaneous flap, in other words the lower belly was moved up to recreate breasts.) Chemotherapy and radiation therapy followed. One year later, I am a survivor!

A   **What happens when an attitude**
Is seasoned full of gratitude,
A dash of courage, a pinch of cheer?
We face the future with no fear!

Attitude is everything! I know when some people hear a cancer diagnosis, they ask, "Why me**??**"

I (the English teacher) said, "Why me**!!**" What a difference an attitude of gratitude makes. I sought the learning experience of the cancer journey and found it daily.

Across my classroom wall are the German words, *"Es lernt niemand aus, bis das Grab ist unser Haus."* (We don't stop learning until we die.) At the start of my 26th school year in the Buffalo district, a doubting student questioned my belief in that statement. "Mrs. Heyerdahl, " Jon asked, "Do you *really* think you can learn something every day?" "Every day!" I assured him.

On the cancer journey, the learning experience was not always pleasant, but I was in excellent company. In Matthew 28:20 God promised to never leave us. "...and lo, I am with you always, even to the end of the age." If I ever felt alone, it was because *I* had drawn away from God. I thank the Lord Jesus for daily lessons; He is my **Almighty Instructor**!

> **"My hair got much much thinner,**
> **some people were appalled**
> **Chemo has a side effect**
> **of making patients bald."**

Nose hairs are an important part of the body! Oh how I once took mine for granted. Chemotherapy gave me a genuine **appreciation** for nose hairs. I gained **awareness** for physical well being, or lack thereof! When my nose began to drip without warning, I carried a tissue constantly. When my eyelashes no longer existed to protect my eyes, I wore glasses. When brushing my teeth triggered my gag reflex, I adjusted the way I spit! When I experienced heartburn for the first time in my 45 years of life, I ate Pepcid-AC like candy.

As a teacher, I *monitor and adjust* in my classroom often; on the cancer journey, I did so also. I believe the words from Philippians 4:13, "I can do all things through Him who strengthens me!" Yes, with God, I was able to **appreciate** the journey through cancer treatment; I gained a deeper **awareness** of just how precious life is.

B   "My hair is much much thinner,
            do not be appalled
      Chemo has a side effect
            of making patients bald.
      It's a temporary crown
            that cancer patients wear.
      I *had* to break the school's rule
            and wear a hat for hair!"

When my hair began to fall out on the seventeenth day after the first chemotherapy treatment, I decided to release it outside to nature. I stepped outside, ran my fingers through my thick blonde hair, gathered clumps between my fingers and tossed the hair in the air, offering it to the birds as construction material for their autumn nests. This action made me feel somewhat in control of this unavoidable situation.

The unconditional love of family and friends made the transition to **bald** much less traumatic. My sister Tammy accompanied me to wig shop at the American Cancer Society. The ACS employee assisting us was entertained by our visit. I tried wigs of black and red and blonde, long and short, straight and curly.

Loving dramatic flare, I changed my personality with each wig. Dear Tammy managed to snap a few pictures of me. We especially enjoyed the long curly locks of red that inspired me to pose with a shoulder bared as I chanted, "I'm too sexy for my body!"

Two dear colleagues from school presented me with a

computer program to help me foresee my baldness and then to plan ahead for a new hairstyle after chemotherapy. This was a gift of love that continues to be a blessing as I share it with others.

> **"The battle belongs to the Lord,"**
> **many have heard me say**
> **"I'm caught in the crossfire,"**
> **God is with me all the way.**

The day after the incision biopsy, I stopped at Mom's for a brief visit. On my way out the door, I mentioned I would be calling the surgeon the next day to get the results. I had an appointment to see him the day after that, but I wanted to know the results as soon as he knew! Mom thought I should wait until I was in his office to hear the report. Even before I heard the diagnosis of cancer, I told my mother, "The **battle** belongs to the Lord." I believed that. He is a mighty warrior! As I drove away in my car... *not one minute later*, what song came on the radio? "The **Battle** Belongs to the Lord!" At the first church service after my surgery, the praise and worship time began with "The **Battle** Belongs to the Lord!" Coincidence? God's voice!

God keeps His promises: the **battle** is His!

C   **"Chemo hasn't been easy, it hasn't been fun**
         But Praise the Lord! I am now done!"

"**Chemotherapy** is NOT for wimps!" was an e-mail I received from another survivor. Amen! I was not a wimp, I could do this! To help see myself through the eight treatments, I visualized the course of my **chemotherapy** to be a baseball diamond. Two down...I was on first base, half done...second base; after number five: wave at the shortstop on the way to third base! What a victory with that eighth treatment to finally reach home plate! I focused on the glory, and my attitude of gratitude kept me in the game.

D   What happens when our attitude
          Is seasoned with some gratitude...
       A dash of courage and some cheer?
          We face our *doctors* with no fear!

The cancer diagnosis widened my circle of acquaintances to include many other cancer patients and numerous members of the medical staff.

I was blessed with exceptional medical care. My goal was to always let these "angels" know how much I appreciated them. A basketful of candy bars accompanied these words to the hospital:

A month has passed since I was your guest;
    My recovery has been the very best.
I'm writing this now for I must share
    How much I appreciated the GREAT care.
The nurses I met on fourth floor east
    Were angels...at the very least!
Dawn, Karen, Sue, Alice and Katie
    Each one is a special lady.
Erica, Betsy, and the names I don't recall:
    You made my stay the best of all.
Room 476 was warmer than toast,
    Yet each helped me to like it the most.
The night I passed out on my husband's belly
    Katie and Alice took care of me as "jelly."
Onto the bed they transferred me QUICKLY.
    One transfusion later, I was no longer sickly.
I'm so pleased with all who cared for me
    Especially Doctors DeAngelis and Ose.
Their nurses and interns also were great
    The Methodist staff gets an A+ rate!
I'm so glad to have been your guest
    In God's Hands, I AM BLESSED!

A month after surgery, I started chemotherapy.

When I first met my oncologist, I sensed no bond, no human relation. What could I do to make that connection happen? An article in a magazine answered my question. Treat her like a person! Ask about her family! Create conversation. Does she enjoy cooking? Will she be home for

Christmas? Smile in the exam room! Chat! Be good to the **doctor**. This has made all the difference.

(I'm sure she enjoyed the bagel at lunch time, the morning muffin, the Swiss chocolate and then the pink rose of gratitude to celebrate the end of my chemotherapy! I look forward to future check-ups, and I suspect she does, too!)

E   Mirror, mirror, who's that I see? Is that reflection really me?

Who was that girl in the mirror? I grew accustomed to my bald reflection, but when the Taxotere took my **eyelashes** and **eyebrows**, I was bumming. The change in my appearance suddenly seemed so drastic. Only humor could help me cope with my tarnished vanity. I pretended to count the remaining lashes, sixteen on one eye, eighteen on the other. Humor can mask and heal! Mascara was no longer a budgetary need! Save the cost of eyebrow waxing! There *were* positives in even this situation!

One year after diagnosis, on the first anniversary of my survival, my hair, **eyelashes** and **eyebrows** had already grown back. The **effects** of chemotherapy were temporary and tolerable. I can hardly remember the details of "chemo days" without reminders, like this **e-mail** I had sent to a friend in Florida during my treatment:

> Today is Thanksgiving, and I am truly thankful for life. God is my Almighty Tour Guide, and 1999 has been a scenic journey! As I've ventured down Chemo Trail, there have been eight excursions. Seven are done, the last one is set for December 6...1:30 to be exact! God has protected me from SO much. I have not suffered as so many have. The doctor ordered me to go on leave until January, so I've been home since October. I feel quite different. The chemo treatments are spaced three weeks apart, and the chemicals take time to run through

my system. I'm ten days out of the last I.V. drip, and normalcy has not returned yet. Aches, pains, dry mouth, taste buds that don't work, so many small changes. My hair is growing back.... slowly. I resemble a concentration camp victim now, and have a whole new empathy for those souls. As I went for the last treatment (#7), I prayed for many things...an acceptable white count so I could get the treatment, NO flu shot, and that the Lord would speak to me through the doctor and nurse. Bottom line: the doctor told me there would be no need to schedule bone or CT scans after #8, because there is no reason to believe any cancer is left! Praise God! I have said from the start, The battle belongs to the Lord! He is my Almighty Physician. I am healed in His name!

F   **"He sends me wonderful angels
in family and in friends.
Cards, meals, phone calls,
His love never ends."**

My hospital room was a busy place during my stay. Each and every guest was medicinal, but Adrianna was extra-special. Her daddy was once my neighbor and student. Adrianna was born just three weeks before my surgery. As a parent, I remember being extremely protective of my **firstborn**. For Wade and Michelle to bring their precious new baby to visit me in the oncology ward was a genuine gift of love. Throughout my chemo and radiation, Adrianna brightened many of my days with her visits.

The day I arrived home from the hospital, I gingerly settled into a chair in the family room. My abdomen was SO tender!

Soon a telephone call came from my **friend** Lilly in Switzerland. Concern for my health caused her to change her RSVP for our daughter's upcoming wedding. She *would* be coming! The emotions within me strained my sutures; was I laughing or crying? How loved I felt to know she would be arriving in two weeks.

Lilly's visit was better than any prescription on the market.

I have never met a more generous man than my **father**. If I give him something, he returns the giving in triplicate. When a snowstorm threatened to keep me home from a radiation treatment, I called Sista Tammy for advice. Who could I ask to drive me to the hospital? Who could best maneuver on the slippery roads? With Tammy's coaxing, I called Dad. How could I ask him for yet another favor? I felt that I owed him so much already! He was *always* helping me, yet without a moment's hesitation he was ready, willing and able to drive to Methodist. We arrived at the hospital safe *and* early!

The love of **family and friends** made me strong. I can never thank them enough.

G   **"No way can I ever forget**
     All the dear people I have met:
From the set-up day and the smile of Robin's
     To daily chats with Natalie Dobbins,
Wonderful people, compassionate folks
     Tender employees who laughed at my jokes.
28 treatments went by so fast;
     The positive staff made it a blast!"

Radiation therapy treatments were daily, Monday through Friday, for six weeks. The treatment itself took less than ten minutes, but the drive time was almost two hours. How would I survive this drudgery?

On the day of my first treatment, I noticed an older gentleman in the waiting room, already dressed in a hospital robe and **gown**. After changing into my "radiation wear," I said to the older man, "We must shop at the same store; we're dressed alike!" Spark! A friendship was kindled. Each day when I arrived, I'd try to match Loren by dressing in a gown and robe of the same printed fabric as his choice of the day. We took pictures of us, the "matching twins!"

When Loren **graduated** from his treatments, his **gift** from me was monogrammed "radiation wear!" When I completed radiation, Loren came back to present me with a plaque of Completion from the Sunshine Salon!

Relationships make all the difference! Yes, **God** loves people more than anything. Is it any wonder how much people can help us on our journey?

H   "He sends me wonderful angels in family
         and in friends.
      Cards, meals, phone calls, His love never ends."

Just when I thought I knew my **husband** Steve, he showed me new depths of his love! When I needed a blood transfusion after surgery, he moved in a cot and stayed "watch" in my room. (I fell asleep, but he observed each drop of blood drip into me!)

My sister Debbie drove me home from the hospital in her smooth-riding van, but Steve was in our driveway waving me a "Welcome Home!"

I was discharged from the hospital with drain tubes and bandages still intact, and Steve was the one who emptied the bottles and changed the dressings. When my white count plummeted and neupogen injections were prescribed, my husband became my home health care provider. I could not tolerate giving myself the shots, so he offered. What a wonderful man God chose for me!

Months after the surgery we were watching a movie, and I became emotional when an actress portraying a cancer patient asked, "Is a woman less of a woman without her breasts and uterus?" Sensing my tears, he grabbed my hand and asked, "Are you okay?" and in doing so, he gave me strength.

His phone calls to "check on me" have brought sun-shine to stormy days after surgery and chemotherapy. After the final reconstruction surgery, when I was sup-posed to be recovering I became overeager with the yard-work and got the lawnmower stuck in the swamp! Steve's reaction? Total compassion! We left the John Deere in the swamp overnight and went out for dinner!

Indeed! "Love bears all things!" I Corinthians 13:7

I   **The incision biopsy path report came back
        and then I heard
        "Lobular carcinoma,"....cancer, in a word.**

The emotions one experiences after hearing the diag-nosis of cancer are novel, unique, unforgettable. I first heard the words "lobular carcinoma" on a Wednesday afternoon. The next day my husband and I met with a sur-geon and nurse, and more appointments were scheduled for Friday morning, beginning at 9:30.

Sleep eluded me both Wednesday and Thursday nights. Early Friday morning, as I struggled with what the substitute teacher would tell my advisory group, I had a brainstorm! I could go to school for the first twenty min-utes and tell the students the diagnosis myself! There would still be plenty of time for me to return home, meet Steve and drive to the radiologist on time.

I woke Steve to tell him my plan. He didn't try to talk me out of it, so I got ready for school and drove into town. As I parked the car in front of school, I suddenly asked myself, "What am I doing? What *will* I tell the kids?" The answer came at that exact moment through a song on the radio. God's timing IS perfect. He spoke through Kathy Troccoli as she sang,

> "Some called Him a prophet. Some called Him a saint. Some couldn't believe their eyes or the words He had to say. Some called Him crazy; some thought he was strange, but I have felt His touch,

and I'll never be the same. I call Him Love. I call Him Mercy. I called Him out of my darkness and pain and He answered my need. I call Him Love. I call Him Healing. He is the One who has filled me with hope and restored life to me. I call Him Love."

Tears streamed from my eyes as I raised my hands to praise my Lord for His presence. I knew He would give me the words to inform my students. Just then I sensed I was being watched. Another teacher walking past my car perhaps thought a car jacking was in progress...Me with my hands up and crying! I waved to let him know I was fine, finished the song, wiped my tears and boldly went in to tell my Prime Time, the advisory group, what was happening. The "peace that passes all understanding" was present. Twenty minutes later, I left with their power ... their power of prayer!

The next week I met with two of my English classes one morning before leaving for more appointments at the clinic. On the whiteboard I had written the daily lesson plan, which included "summer homework." Groans were audible as soon as students read the board. "Come on, what summer homework, Mrs. Heyerdahl?" I assured them that not all would have to do it. The homework was a special request I was making of those who believed in Jesus. I asked them to pray for my healing.

Two months later I received a card from Ryan who wrote, "I wanted you to know I am doing my summer homework."

Inspiration may come from kids or adults, family, friends or strangers, a book or the radio; if we listen, we will hear!

J   "The plan was not to miss much school
            But cancer treatment was not cool.
        I ended up down on my knees
            Asking, "Father, help me please!
        You know whom the students need."
            And He gave us Mrs. Mead.
        She has been absolutely great
            Teaching classes of English 8.
        Committed she is, beyond measure.
            Compassion she has; what a treasure!
        I'm so thankful for Jackie dear;
            What a difference she's made this year!"

I was determined that chemo would *not* keep me away from school. The school year began just after I received the third of eight treatments. "If I have to miss any days," I told the Personnel Director, "God will provide the right person to be in my room." I spoke in faith when I said, "God already knows who will be in my room each day of the school year."

How true those words were! When I was forced to stay home full time for three months and half time for two more months, God provided Jackie, alias "Super Sub!" She stepped into my classroom and taught with love and devotion. We worked as a team, God, **Jackie** and Jan!

K   After chemo was done I had one month to
            get stronger
        Then I underwent radiation therapy,
            six weeks longer.
        28 trips to Methodist Hospital, oh! what a ride!
        Once again the Lord was there, drivers to provide.
        Not a single day did I have to drive alone.
        God knows the needs of those He has called
            His own!

Kindness is volunteering to drive a cancer patient to radiation treatment. Oh the kindness I received! Before I even knew the date when radiation would begin, **Karla** said she wanted to start a calendar and get "pencilled in!"

Someone did indeed drive me EVERY day for all six weeks! Dad filled in at the last minute *twice* because of nasty wintry weather. Mom was the Monday driver for the first four weeks. Angelic friends that God truly provided took care of all, yes, ALL the other days! Indeed, "He knows the needs of those He has called His own!"

Karla frequently talks about "random acts of kindness" in her motivational speaking engagements. She truly "walks that talk." Her plan for my final day of radiation therapy was to drive separately to the hospital (as a surprise) and be on the table when I went in for treatment. Another commitment forced her to go with Plan B...she sent a basket of phenomenal treasures in the trunk of my sister Tammy's car. I exited the last radiation therapy into a room of flowers, friends, family, and Karla's basket. In it she had notes attached to the *treasures*. "WATCH YOUR HAIR GROW" on the mirror. "We have reason to make music!" on the harmonica. "Use these now, CELEBRATE" on bubbles. "Your future's so bright, you gotta wear shades" on sunglasses strategically placed on a HOPE beanie bear. The basket was overflowing with her love and the special touch of a survivor's empathy.

There are times when only a survivor can calm a cancer patient. God **kindly** kindled my friendship with **Karla**, and she has given me strength. Thanks, Girlfriend!

L   **"He sends me wonderful angels
in family and in friends.
Cards, meals, phone calls,
His love never ends."**

The day after I completed radiation therapy, a beautiful bouquet of flowers was delivered to my classroom with a note of congratulations from my family. Minutes later, I received this e-mail **letter** of **love**:

Mom,

I just wanted to let you know how proud I am of you for making it through these past nine months. You were so brave and faithful. I love you very much and am so very glad that everything turned out the way that it has...all for the best! You were the best example of bravery, optimism and faith that I have ever seen. Congratulations and ... I LOVE YOU!

I had just returned to teach half-days when the following e-mail **letter** of **love** arrived from a former student whom I hadn't seen in about three years!

Dear Mrs. Heyerdahl,

There has been much thought given to whether or not I should write you. I do not wish to be a nuisance or to pry. My heart has been with you since that last week of school last year when I heard of your situation. I figure using this form of technology, e-mail, you can delete this message if you feel it's obtrusive and need not reply.

I have been helping out with the Middle School play. There I have heard much about you and the students' reaction to what's happening. The first thing I realized is that there are many out there that adore you as I do. The very first thing anyone said to me (before I was introduced even) was whether or not I had you as an eighth grade English teacher...and to proudly announce that you were back in school that day (Monday). You've touched them. Even the boys. Even people not in your classes. It takes a REAL teacher to do that. Especially when you're going through a tough time yourself. You are my role model. Not only as a teacher, but also as a person. I love how you relate to teenagers. You have not forgotten what it was to be one. That is my goal…to reach out to students as you do.

I believe that God made you extra specially. Cancer is part of the journey God has set for you, only because He knows you are strong enough for it. And along the way you can teach a life-lesson to your students about the strength of the soul and the power of faith.

Your student always,
Missy

As I underwent chemotherapy during the school year, my students gained a novel learning experience. A few of them shared **letters** at the end of the year. Erin wrote,

"You not only taught me English, but you taught me about the real meaning of life. Almost every day leaving your class I had something new to think about. I look up to you so much. The way you always have a smile and great attitude toward everything just makes you a great role model and a great person to admire. To me I see you as an angel, God spent a little more time with you!"

Kayla moved me to tears when I read her words:

"I know you have changed a lot of lives for the best, you have changed my life! Everything you said I listened so carefully to understand it. I have not gotten along with some of the kids in this class, and gotten into fights with some of them…but when we read the novel at the end of the year and you talked about holding grudges and forgiveness, I realized that you were 100% right, and in my heart I forgave everyone, and hoped they forgave me. I just can't thank you enough, for everything. I loved hearing your stories and all the funny experiences

you had. God put you here in my life for a special reason. You will always be my role model...
P.S. I hope my sister gets you, she will love you as much as I do!"

Lisabeth encouraged me with this e-mail a week after surgery:

You really are my GODmother. You help me keep my focus on Him. You live your faith, which is the best testimony anybody could ever give. I remember all those special bonding times we've had...

You gave me the first flowers I ever got...yellow daffodils from the American Cancer Society, when I was six or seven years old. Beautiful!

...it was so cool when I got to stay overnight at your house on a school night. One time you packed me a cold lunch, which was a very rare and therefore special thing for me, and you even let me put pop in it. All you had was Diet Pepsi, which I didn't like, but I took it anyway. When I tried to open it at lunch that day, it exploded all over. :-)

Then, of course, Junior High. Whoa, awesome. Yep! Mrs. Heyerdahl, the best teacher in the world is MY auntie!... You really love your job and life and God and you let it all show in your personality and teaching style and everything you do.

...so many memories I have... They make me smile. :-) Thanks for all the memories and the ones that are to come!

Love you so much Godmom

Doesn't that Bible say ...WE SHALL OVER-COME BY THE BLOOD OF THE LAMB!!!!

Yay for Jesus! He's our Healer!

M   **"The battle belongs to the Lord"**
       many have heard me say.
       I'm caught in the crossfire,
       God is with me all the way!

Who could ever imagine all the **medicine** a cancer patient could be introduced to in six months? Cytoxan, Adriamicin, Taxotere, Neupogen, Tamoxifen, not to mention Endocet, Torecan, Allegra, Deltasone, Pepcid AC, Tums, Rolaids, and more! I stood firm on my motto, "The battle belongs to the Lord." Each treatment I received, every medication I took, I offered to God as a weapon in His battle.

As a mom, I would never send my children off to school without the supplies they needed. How could I *not* give my Lord the weapons available for the battle? I underwent chemotherapy for the Lord, offering it to Him as a weapon in His battle. During each radiation session, I prayed for God to guide and control the radiation; His omniscient eyes could see where He needed the rays.

Even now as I am taking Tamoxifen, as I swallow each pill, I pray that it may be a weapon for God in His battle, and I declare Him victorious and glorious!

N   **What happens when our attitude
Is seasoned with some gratitude…
A dash of courage and some cheer?
We face our *nurses* with no fear!**

Park Nicollet Clinic assigned me to Robin Lally, Breast Care **Nurse** upon my initial diagnosis. Robin offered me her wisdom, her ear, her shoulder and her pager number! My experiences from diagnosis through treatments were far from typical; poison ivy, a bee sting, a car accident, and hives are not the norm. Robin's responses to the many pages were prompt and professional. Having a rapport with the medical personnel adds to the healthiness of the treatment.

I tried to let each member of the medical staff know I was appreciative and grateful. This was a thank you after the final **nipple** reconstruction:

Gratitude to the Plastic Surgeon and Nurse

In the past year, I've seen many changes
    for the better, not for the worse.
It's time to thank Dr. DeAngelis and Paula,
    his blessed nurse.
When I first met these two in 1999,
    the month was May,
After a diagnosis of "lobular carcinoma,"
    I came to hear what they would say.
With calming reassurance
    and a voice reflecting peace,
Paula had me watch a video, yes!
    a TRAM flap release.
She apologized for not having popcorn
    then started the cassette.
My sister Debbie joined me
    just as my eyes were getting wet.
Knowing I was about to make a major decision soon
With confidence Dr. DeAngelis, entered the room.
Choosing words I understood,
    he further explained the TRAM flap
And then with his artistic pen, he diagrammed a "map!"
The scheduling was miraculous
    when God created eight hours of slack
The calendar of the surgeons had
    two cancellations, back to back.
The surgery was successful, and oh was I in luck
To get both a breast reduction and a tummy-tuck!
Such a perfect new belly button on me
    the doctor did make
That no one will believe me when I say it is a fake!
After chemo was completed and radiation, too,
I returned to Dr. DeAngelis...his finishing work to do.
Creating new nipples to some may seem vain or quirky
But this was his job, and he even made them perky!
He fulfilled my every wish, because I know he cares
And my new nipples are perfect without any hairs!
Yes, I'm a satisfied patient and wanted them to know
How much they are appreciated. Now I've told them so!

O   "The wedding was beautiful...
          I attended! I was able!
     I even fulfilled our daughter's wish
          and danced on the table!"

The night before our daughter's wedding, I hardly slept. Yet, the day of the wedding I had abundant energy and was told I looked radiant. (Yeah, God!)

Just before midnight, I was mingling with guests when my son and niece escorted me by my elbows to the table where my husband was seated, near the dance floor. As we approached the table, my son pulled out a chair and gestured for me to use it as a stairway to my "tabletop dance floor!" Without missing a beat, I stepped up and then danced **on the table**. The words of the song were music to my ears and to my heart! "I will survive! I will survive! I've got so much life to live; I've got so much love to give. I will survive!"

Eleven months later, I participated with six family members in the Race for the Cure. As a survivor, I received one of the pink T-shirts, which was imprinted: *"I will survive! I've got so much life to live; I've got so much love to give."*

Sometimes God's voice is so **obvious**!

P   "I must also tell of the miracle
          when God used a little poodle
     From the pup I got poison ivy,
          oh that stuff is brutal!
     I ended up on medicine that was truly fine.
     It elevated my blood levels in a way divine.
     I qualified for a cancer study,
          Why would this seem strange?
     The meds for the poison ivy
          put my blood counts in the range!
     The nurse tried to say the counts
          were *artificially* elevated
     The correct word was *divinely*,
          to her I simply stated!"

After my diagnosis, I prayed that I would be allowed to participate in a Breast Cancer Study so the results of my case would go into the national pool of information and perhaps benefit other women with similar cases. The oncologist explained that my blood counts would determine if I could participate, and she added that both my hemoglobin and white counts were low.

Two weeks after surgery, and one week before our daughter's wedding, my family celebrated Father's Day at a lake cabin. I thoroughly enjoyed the company of my sister's poodle, Kala. The next day, however, I suspected the pooch was to blame for the **poison ivy** on my arm. As Mom was driving me into the clinic, I began to feel overwhelmed with frustration.

Wasn't cancer surgery enough? Chemo was about to begin... WHY **poison ivy**, dear God, why? I heard His voice, "Trust Me." In my heart I wondered, "Trust You for poison ivy?" Yet... I did. The prescribed Medrol pack cleared up the **poison ivy** before the wedding.

The next week I had blood tests to determine if I could participate in the Study Group. I trusted God, and He used a poodle to help me qualify! The medicine was a steroid, and in clearing up the poison ivy, my blood counts became temporarily elevated. The nurse called this elevation "artificial," but I know it was "divine!"

Q   **What thing about this journey
has been the very best?
I have nestled in with God
and found His special rest!**

One of my favorite prayers to God has been, "Lord, I want to know Your will, please hit me over the head so I know it." Ah the blessed bruises! "Ask and you shall receive!" (Matthew 7:7) God keeps His promises!

I like to begin each day reading a number of devotionals. When the same scripture appeared within days, I sensed a "bruise" and the **Q** word for this book! The words of scripture are in Mark 6:31. "Come aside...and rest a while." The devotional asked, "Are you running at full speed? Let up on the throttle." The second one said, "If you're weary from your labors in the valley, the Lord may be saying to you, "Come aside... and rest a while."

The journey through chemotherapy and radiation brought me to a **quiet** time with Jesus. I prayed more, and I praised Him more. I rested, and He restored my soul. Thank you, Lord.

R   Radiation therapy is now over and done...
But memories will keep alive the fun!
No way can I ever forget
All the dear people I have met:
From the set-up day and the smile of Robin's
To daily chats with Natalie Dobbins,
Wonderful memories, compassionate folks
Tender employees who laughed at my jokes.
28 treatments went by so fast
The positive staff made it a blast!
Mondays were good but could have been great
If I never had to reveal my weight!
Thank you for tolerance, dear nurse Grace,
The scale is a monster I can hardly face.
Dr. Haselow knows all about the trick
When I topped 200 with a lead brick.
Tammy, thanks for the robes the gowns of blue.
Jessica, Erin, and Camie, you are wonderful, too!
To each and every member of the radiation staff:
Keep up the great work! Continue to laugh!
Oh what a pleasure I have had as your guest
To say the very least, I have been blessed.

P.S. We cannot forget the best of the snickers:
Creative Wednesdays with silly stickers!

Radiation therapy was the "piece of cake" that so many told me it would be. I added a bit of frosting to it on Wednesdays when I wore stickers for nipples. The technicians had never experienced a sense of humor like mine. The collection of stickers included smiley faces, giraffes saying "Stand Proud," winking faces, red circles declaring "I Voted" and gold sequined tassels for the final day.

Loren returned on that last day, and Debra was there, too. She and I had met during chemo and were now enjoying daily chats in the waiting room. I had to have a picture of Loren, Debra and I together. As I reached my arms back to hug my friends, something hit my foot. One of the tassels fell from my breast! I picked it up and held it in the picture for all to see!

That last day of **radiation** was bittersweet as I said goodbye to the staff and friends, but the **relationships** did not end. When I returned with chocolate treats months later, Natalie still called me by name! Debra and I now chat at home on the phone rather than in the waiting room!

S   The surgeon's scheduler said,
           "Our calendar has no room."
       The Almighty Scheduler acted
           before I could feel gloom!
       He worked a little miracle as soon as I did pray;
       And I was on the table in just over a day

My husband, Steve, and I met with the Surgeon on June 1, six days after my diagnosis. Our decision was made! I would undergo a bilateral mastectomy with a TRAM flap. Dr. Ose warned me that I would need three weeks for recovery. Fine. Our daughter's wedding was 25 days away! My surgery would require an eight-hour time slot, coordinating the schedules of the surgeon, the plastic surgeon and the operating room. The surgeon escorted us to Susan, the scheduler. She opened the calendar; it was fully booked for two weeks. She offered to pencil me in for June 17.

I spoke in faith, "The Almighty **Scheduler** already has this on paper, He just hasn't shown us." Susan's reaction was one of uncertainty, to say the least. Steve and I left without a surgery date. Before I returned home though, Susan had left a message for me to call her. I did.

She said, "Jan, the freakiest thing happened. Two back-to-back surgeries cancelled for the day after tomorrow. Can you be at the hospital by 6 AM?"

I assured her that I would be there; then I went on to explain that this was not "freaky," this was *God*. I reminded her of my words, "The Almighty **Scheduler** already has this on paper, He just hasn't shown us."

Siblings

When had I last danced with my sisters? Songs of praise inspired us to dance before the Lord our Maker. Cancer turned us closer to God, drew us closer to each other. I am blessed with four sisters and a brother. Each one had a special part in my healing process.

Sister Debbie

Sister Debbie should receive a Postmaster Award for having sent me the most cards! Repeatedly, she heard God's voice and knew what I needed to hear. One of my favorite cards was signed with a paw print of Kala the poodle! (Remember? The one in the patch of poison ivy!)

Another favorite that earned a spot on the front of the frig was a circular postcard with a bald stick person proclaiming, "Who needs hair anyway!"

Debbie's precious phone calls and inspirational cards and e-mails kept me in check with the Lord. I'm forever grateful.

Sister Joyce

Sister Joyce has major health needs of her own, yet she poured her loving support on me repeatedly. I'm forever grateful.

Sister Judy

Three of the five girls in my family are teachers. Judy understood the difficult time I had staying home, away from students, for three months. After my final chemo, I visited her classroom to share the coloring book that Karla and I had narrated. Judy allowed me to instruct the students in an art project with the rubber stamps I'd brought from home. The students later shared their gratitude in beautiful card creations. Three different sets of cards arrived from Judy's classroom throughout my cancer treatments. I'm forever grateful.

Brother Larry and Sister-in-law Judy

Not a week passed during chemotherapy that I did not receive a note from my brother and sister-in-law's church letting me know they were praying for me. I felt the power of prayer, as I never had before! I'm forever grateful.

Sister Tammy

Tammy and I are ten years apart in age, but there are days when our hearts beat as one. As I look back, I realize Tammy was with me from "day one" when we scheduled our mammograms "back-to-back" in March. Yes, from the beginning, she was there with me.

She phoned me at school on the morning of what would be diagnosis day to ask what time I would be calling the doctor for the report on the biopsy. She persisted until I finally told her I was calling from school at 4:30. That's when Tammy arrived! We were together when Dr. Ose told me the biopsy showed lobular carcinoma.

As I told him our daughter's wedding was exactly one month away, he advised me to not wait until after the wedding! As he spoke, I scripted his words so Tammy knew his part of the conversation. After making arrangements to see him first thing the next morning, I hung up the phone and quoted a line from a book I had recently read, "I think God overdid it."

Tammy and I hugged and cried, then I called my pastor. I requested prayer for my Steve as I went home to tell him. Tammy went home to explore the websites that could help me make an informed decision.

Tammy took me to all ten chemo appointments. (I received only eight treatments, but was sent home twice, delayed because of low blood counts.) We always "packed up" for the treatments: CD player, Kathy Troccoli's song, other Christian music, my blanket from Ruth and my book of all the doctor and lab reports.

The chemotherapy drugs made me forgetful for days. Why do the nurses start telling the information about the meds AFTER administering them? I had no train of thought! Tammy listened, though, and she remembered.

The first day of workshop for school was three days after chemo #3. I woke up nauseous. Just as I sat down at the kitchen table with my book of information to figure out which medication I should take, the telephone rang; it was Tam. No reading necessary! Tammy told me what to take. The chemo didn't effect her memory! God spoke; she listened and made the telephone call.

After having the second and third treatments delayed, I was anxious for the fourth and hopeful it would be on time. Tammy and I arrived at the clinic just as I was scheduled for the lab. I checked in then rushed to the bathroom, telling Tammy she could give blood if my name was called. I knew for sure that I would qualify for a treatment if I could use her blood counts. As I walked back into the waiting room, Tammy was coming out of the lab, holding a cotton ball and tape on her arm. I was impressed! She was such a trooper to even do the blood draw for me! Seconds later the lab technician stepped out and invited me in. I'd been had! It was a phony blood draw.

Not to worry...I did qualify, and I did it with my own blood!

Tammy added humor to yet another doctor visit by prompting the nurse to place her foot on the scale for my regular weigh-in. Unsuspecting at first, I was baffled. How could I have gained ten pounds? Wait! (Weight!) I see a foot on the back of the scale. You are busted, Nurse Ian! Very funny, Tammy!

We took pictures at every chemo session, and what a joy to reflect on those bygone days. My favorite was the last one, snapped under the EXIT sign of the Cancer Center! I had my hand on the knob, so the sign was even illuminated, yet our smiles outshone the letters.

Our hearts do beat independently, but mine goes on because of my **sister**, Tammy. Tammy was my most stead-fast support. I'm forever grateful.

T

When the church secretary called to ask if I would share my **testimony** at a Lenten Service, I eagerly consented. To keep within the time allotment, I chose to express myself through poetry:

> I would like to share my faith; this is no baloney.
> Directly from my heart, here's my testimony.
> I was raised in love, attended Sunday School.
> By the time I was 10, I let the Lord rule!
> Jesus Christ moved right into my heart;
> Every single day He has been a vital part.
> As the years have passed
>   His love has been sufficient.
> Our Most Holy God truly is Omniscient.
> He blessed me with my husband, Steve,
>   and we moved to Oakview Lane.
> Then we joined VOG, God's will
>   was clear and plain!
> Since 1976 this church has been our "daybreak;"
> Once we tried a transfer; oops! That was a mistake!
> We were still in Plymouth
>   when Chrissy and Paul were born;
> Now we're off in Buffalo
>   where I'm a teacher, sworn!

My most recent story of the Lord's love so fine
Started just last year in 1999.
Early in the year during a breast self-exam
I felt a change and then had a mammogram.
After more mammograms and an ultrasound
The radiologist said, "Nothing could be found."
Persistent I am and saw another doc in May.
His recommendation,
    "See what a surgeon will say."
The surgeon took needle biopsies, a total of four
The results were "suspicious,"
    so he went back for more.
The incision biopsy path report came back
    and then I heard
"Lobular carcinoma," ....cancer, in a word.
"Oh my!" I responded on that 26th day of May...
"In just one month
    it's our daughter's wedding day!"
Before I had the chance to fret or fear or worry,
I let go to Jesus and He acted in a hurry.
The surgeon's scheduler said,
    "Our calendar has no room."
The Almighty Scheduler acted
    before I could feel gloom!
He worked a little miracle as soon as I did pray;
And I was on the table in just over a day.
Yes! On the third of June I had a blessed 8-hour nap
During a bilateral mastectomy and a TRAM flap.
The recovery was phenomenal,
    as I nestled in God's palm.
How could I relax and smile?
    How could I keep calm?
"The battle belongs to the Lord,"
    many have heard me say,
"I'm caught in the crossfire,"
    God is with me all the way!
I must also tell of the miracle
    when God used a little poodle.
From the pup I got poison ivy,
    oh that stuff is brutal!
I ended up on medicine that was truly fine.
It elevated my blood levels in a way divine.

I qualified for a cancer study,
    why would this seem strange?
The meds for the poison ivy
    put my blood counts in the range!
The nurse tried to say the counts
    were *artificially* elevated
The correct word was *"divinely,"*
    to her I simply stated!
The wedding was beautiful...I attended! I was able!
I even fulfilled our daughter's wish
    and danced on the table!
I completed chemotherapy. Eight done, none to go!
Did I stay home from school last fall? God willing,
    I said NO!
I not only returned to teach my classes of English 8
On Sundays I shepherded Disciple Zone kids,
    they are really great!
My hair was much, much thinner,
    some people were appalled;
Chemo has a side effect of making patients bald.
It's a temporary crown that cancer patients wear
I broke the school's rule and wore a hat for hair!
God blessed me in Disciple Zone
    when DJ asked of me
"Would you take off your wig, so we could all see?"
His words were such a blessing,
    they spoke loud and clear
Of Christian acceptance, one doesn't need hair here!
After chemo was done
    I had one month to get stronger
Then I underwent radiation therapy,
    six weeks longer.
28 trips to Methodist Hospital,
    oh! what a ride!
Once again the Lord was there, drivers to provide.
Not a single day did I have to drive alone.
God knows the needs of those
    He has called His own!
He sent me wonderful angels
    in family and in friends.
Cards, meals, phone calls, His love never ends.
I'm thankful for the chance
    to be showered with such love;

My praise and thanksgiving go
    to the Almighty Healer above.
Some people asked me...
    how did you survive so well?
Was it your clinic? Your faith? Your attitude?
    Please do tell!
The Lord Jesus Christ
    has provided my every single need.
Is that my "final answer?" Yes it is, indeed!
Every day God gives us a chance to show how we
    Either *bitter* or *better* will make our lives to be.
I praise God I'm *better* in His Arms.
Try it and you'll see, Life loses its alarms!

U   The journey I experienced I will not soon forget
    More important than the journey
        are the friends I have met
    Cancer survivors share a bond,
        for girls: a sisterhood...
    "Been there, done that;" we have *understood!*

My grandmother died two weeks after I completed radiation therapy. At the funeral, a lady from Grandma's church told me I looked like "a million dollars." I was surprised to hear this from a woman I did not recognize. She introduced herself, and I vaguely knew the family name; her daughter had graduated a year ahead of me in high school. As the conversation continued, the lady told me her daughter, Diane, was living on the East Coast and undergoing eight treatments for breast cancer; she had just received number five. I left the funeral with plans to contact Diane.

The plan was God-inspired. Diane was on the same chemotherapy as I had received. She had just experienced the same horrific pain after the fifth cycle. Her doctor said it wasn't normal. I told her it was! Through prayer, e-mail, phone calls and cards I sent her strength. (I **understood**!)

She replied:

Dear Jan,

I FINISHED MY LAST CHEMO! I wore a lime green shirt, lime green Capri's (I tell my daughter we called them pedal pushers!), a tropical wrap of lime green, hot orange, hot turquoise, and hot pink. Huge hot pink earrings and a hot pink tropical necklace. However, this was too dull for me. I added my daughter's dance top hat, which is solid gold sequins! Everyone had a good laugh. A gold sequin top hat looks mighty fine on a bald head!

I loved your picture and card. I laughed and felt that sisterhood only we can feel. Thank you for being my friend. Thank you for pulling me through! Onward to surgery and radiation (will I glow in the dark?)

...Thanks for being there for me. I send you wishes of sunshine and friendship.

Love, Diane

V   **The incision biopsy path report came back and then I heard "Lobular carcinoma,"...cancer, in a word.**

"Lobular carcinoma" sounded big, but I knew God was bigger. I learned to never let Satan attack through **vocabulary** words! God will translate anything, anytime.

Chemotherapy and **vanity** are not friends. Looking in the mirror could ruin a day for me, so I avoided my reflection.

Phone calls from Mom were always high points in my day because she knew how I was feeling. Moms know.

Even today, months after my last treatment, weeks after my first haircut, she still closes our phone conversation with "Good bye, Beautiful." When I least felt it, Mom spoke it!

Moms know!

W   **"Thank you for tolerance, dear nurse Grace,
The scale is a monster I can hardly face.
Dr. Haselow knows all about the trick
When I topped 200 with a lead brick."**

Who steps on the scale more than obstetrics patients? Oncology patients. I schemed and found a way to deal with the dreaded **weigh-in**. Before leaving for the clinic, I would step on the scale at home to be sure I had not gained or lost a significant amount of weight. At the clinic I humored the staff as I stepped on the scale with my purse on my shoulder, a book in my hand, a coat over my arm. The nurse simply shrugged and recorded the weight. Unknown to the staff, my secret goal was to top the scale at 200 by carrying as much as possible! The day I succeeded, the nurse was gone, and the doctor politely recorded my weight at 216.2, then I showed him a surprise: a lead brick under my robe. Laughter from a doctor is medicinal! Humor heals! The radiation staff was "the best of the best!"

Wright County has a Breast Cancer Support Group that meets in Monticello about eight times a year. My initial visit convinced me that I WILL return.

The agenda for next month includes a game of Breast BINGO. One of the survivors inquired, "Will there be a booby prize?" Indeed! "A merry heart doeth good like a medicine!" Proverbs 17:22

My heart was quite serious when two days after my diagnosis, I wrote these **words** in my journal:

I want to be able to shine for Jesus. My heart aches for the children whose parents do not believe and therefore deprive their kids of church. Use me, Lord, as You have never used me before. Employ me to witness!

Words are so powerful. A very dear friend repeatedly said just two words to me, but they were all I needed from him, "Be strong."

Sometimes we must fight the words we hear. People do not always think before speaking. After chemo #7, I was back on neupogen to keep my white count up and was therefore able to attend a very special family wedding. I was eleven days out of chemo, which meant my body was at its weakest. I was on Advil, big time; by the time the wedding dance started, I had taken the maximum for the day: twelve.

Many family members were on the dance floor. I was an exhausted spectator, alone at a table, when someone sat down beside me and said, "You look dead; you should go home." Then she walked away.

Numbness ran through me. Tears welled in my eyes. The Holy Spirit took me by the shoulders and shook life into me. I heard a voice, "You are not dead, go dance, Girl, dance! Show her YOU ARE ALIVE!" I obeyed and danced and danced. The energy was from above, not from within! As I danced, my heart became heavy for other chemo patients who might hear words like "You look dead; you should go home, " and might not have the Holy Spirit to comfort them. How could I help? I knew of one way: stop the words!

I left the dance floor to seek out the person who had spoken those words to me. I simply stated, "When you told me 'You look dead; you should go home,' I found those words hurtful and hateful. I'm over it, but I hope you would never say that to another chemo patient." She replied, "I never meant to hurt you."

Words are weapons that can guard and protect, shield and honor, OR injure and kill, maim and destroy. We must choose our **words** with care.

X   **Make Breast Self-Exam a monthly event.**
It will prove to be time well spent.

The importance of a monthly breast self-**exam** is forever on my heart. Four mammograms and two ultrasounds came back clean for me, even though I felt a change in my breast. Persistence paid off when I sought advice from another doctor. I learned the value of listening to my body, following *my* feelings.

Lobular carcinoma is sneaky; machines don't easily detect it.

I've been asked, "What did it feel like? Was it a marble? A pea?" For me, the change was simply firmness, a thickening of tissue, and not a defined shape. I was able to detect the change because I regularly did breast self-exams. By performing monthly breast self-exams, women will know if a change occurs.

Women must boldly be their own advocate, know their bodies and be persistent with doctors!

Y   **My hair was much, much thinner,**
        some people were appalled;
    Chemo has a side effect of making patients bald.

After the second chemotherapy, my wig and I became buddies. Why not name this new friend? I called it **Ydlab**, yes, **Ydlab**, which is "baldy" backwards. **Ydlab** provided great comic relief. My nieces all posed for a picture in it at Thanksgiving dinner.

With long hair I had enjoyed versatility and variety, wearing my hair down or up in French braids, pony tails, twists, etc. I discovered that a wig could offer versatility, too. Some days I wore it backwards! The day I was caught in the rain, I learned that water collects on a wig; run-off is limited. To remove the puddle on my brain, I stepped into the restroom of a restaurant to shake off **Ydlab**. As I put my wig back in place, I discovered a "new do" similar to one resulting from electric shock. Just then another lady entered the restroom. Her face reflected that same electric shock! I wonder if she knew Ydlab was a wig?

> **Here's a little warning of what cancer patients feel**
> **I hope this helps you cope and even makes you heal!**

Yikes! Depression is a telemarketer at a cancer patient's door, constantly nagging. "Buy me! Bottom out! What a deal! Pity party time! Sale! Pout with passion!" **Yikes!** So often the invitations from depression and worry were present.

I resisted with God's help. At a time when I needed to hear these words, they came to me from KTIS: "Worry is the darkroom where the devil takes us to develop negatives." God knows our needs. **Yeah, God!**

Z   **God blessed me in Disciple Zone**
when DJ asked of me
"Would you take off your wig, so we could all see?"
His words were such a blessing,
        they spoke loud and clear
Of Christian acceptance,
        one doesn't need hair here!

Disciple Zone is our Sunday School at church. I "shepherd" a group of fifth and sixth graders, reviewing the weekly Bible lesson, relating it to current times, praying with these children.

At our initial Sunday in September, I was up front with them and explained that I'd had surgery and was undergoing chemo. Did any of them know what chemo was? Mike provided an excellent answer for the class, "Chemotherapy is medicine that kills fast growing cells."

"What are some fast growing cells besides cancer?" I further asked.

Mike replied, "Hair."

I proceeded to explain that the chemo had caused my hair to fall out and I was wearing a wig. DJ raised his hand. "Would you take off your wig so we could see?"

With a smile I revealed my bald head and asked DJ if he realized how much that request meant to me. He had just indirectly told me that I was unconditionally accepted; hair was not needed in **Disciple Zone!**

My niece, Laura, entered Heaven three months before I was diagnosed. As I recovered from surgery, endured chemotherapy and radiation therapy, and finished reconstruction surgery, precious memories of Laura gave me a **zeal** for life!

Laura was born with a special heart, and her heart goes on in each of us who knew her. In the nine and a half years I was her Godmom, she taught me how to trust God and have faith. Laura's thoughts reached beyond mine. When asked who she looked forward to seeing in Heaven, she replied, "Noah and Joseph, you know, the one with the Amazing Technicolor Dreamcoat!"

By the age of five, Laura had set her sights on High. I called one day to tell her mother of the death of another little girl. Laura answered, "Hi Godmom."

"Hi Laura, may I talk to your mother, please?"

"Don't you want to talk to me, Godmom?"

"I'm a little sad right now. Remember the other little girl named Laura that we pray for? She went to be with Jesus today."

Laura exclaimed, "The real Jesus?!"

She was so excited for Laura Swanson to be in Heaven. It is Laura's eagerness, enthusiasm, **zeal** that kept me focused on High!

These were my words for Laura Shadduck's Celebration of Life service:

> **Laura, Godkid, Sweetheart, Friend...**
> **You made the race to the very end!**
> **We know you're now on God's team:**
> **Gymnastics on the floor and beam,**
> **Doing cartwheels, jumps and flips;**
> **Praising Jesus with pink lips,**

Singing to God in worship and praise,
Fully-winded for all your new days.
You've blessed us here with your 9 years
With your faith in Jesus you overcame fears.
Your honesty caught some off guard
Love can sometimes seem quite hard.
We'll miss your vocabulary, your jokes
    and each game
Life without Laura just won't be the same.
Your love for rocking you never outgrew:
Snuggling and singing were favorites, too.
The book on the piano is open to your latest song:
"My heart will go on," How true! How strong!
You touched lives at your school, Cedar Ridge.
From earth to heaven you help us to bridge.
You shared your love at the Church of Jubilee
A clearer picture of Heaven we now can see.
When at last you got your scooter
No one in the neighborhood was cuter.
You were chosen to be the Flower Girl in June...
Looks like you got your wings too soon.
You made us laugh, you made us cry.
Now you make us wonder why?
Why did God need you to be His angel now?
Why couldn't He ten more years allow?
He knew your heart from before your birth;
He knew how long to leave you on this earth.
He saved you from any more pain,
And now you're in His domain.
No more worries! No more cares!
No more looks! No more stares!
You fulfilled the meaning of the name
    Laura: Victorious
And the legacy you leave honors God the Father,
    Glorious!
You were such a special sister to Katie
She is a much more blessed young lady.

Daddy and Mommy prepared you on the ground
and in the sky
Now you have your wings, at last you can fly.
Fly Little Angel, dear Gift of God ...
Your memory forever we will applaud!

I am forever grateful to Laura for inspiring me with her **zeal.**

Conclusion

So now we've shared our ABCs
And of course our LMNOPs.
We offer hope, comfort and praise
To each of you, all of your days.
God is good... all the time
With His help, we'll make the climb.
Affliction can make one stronger, for sure
If with Jesus we choose to endure.
We never stop learning until we die,
So make today an exclamation, "Why!"

Order Form

To purchase additional copies of *The LMNOPs of Surviving Cancer*, please fill out the form below:

Number of books   _____   × $14.95   = _____
Shipping/Handling   per book   ×   2.95   = _____
Sales Tax (MN residents only) per book   ×   .97   = _____
                                                      Total   _____

Ship to:
Name: _____

Address: _____

City: _____ State: _____ Zip: _____

Phone: _____

Make checks payable to: ***Humor Xchange***

If you would like Karla or Jan to insert a personalized message, please include that here:

_____
_____
_____
_____
_____

Mail or fax your order to:

Jan Heyerdahl
700 Hansack Ave. SE
Buffalo, MN 55313-4614
Fax 763-477-5727